"*Unstressed* uses the latest science to show readers how to master their emotions to create a fulfilled life. True contentment is attainable, as Alane Daugherty shows in this wonderful book."

> —**Paul J. Zak, PhD**, professor at Claremont Graduate University, and author of *Trust Factor*

"Such a wonderfully practical book, full of simple, powerful ways to step out of stress and into wholehearted living. Deeply intelligent and immediately useful."

> —**Rick Hanson, PhD**, author of *Resilient*

"*Unstressed* is a skillful guide to managing stress. It is clearly and simply written, and will help the reader develop skills and efficacy. The focus on the body and heart is a unique contribution."

> —**Frederic Luskin, PhD**, senior consultant in wellness at Stanford University School of Medicine, and author of *Forgive for Good*

"*Unstressed* frames stress as the emotional disequilibrium we can all easily recognize in our lives, with ample discoveries from science to explain why, then skillfully applies practices of mindful awareness to recover our inner equilibrium, and carefully designed heart-based practices to fully recover our ease and vitality. A clear and practical road map for reliably moving into resilience and flourishing. A true and timely gift."

> —**Linda Graham, MFT**, author of *Resilience*

"*Unstressed* explains the science and provides the skills for transforming the emotional chaos of stressfulness into resilience and well-being. It describes how mindfulness and heartfulness, working together, cultivate the calm and connection for which we all yearn. When our hearts are erratic with reactivity, this book restores us to the heartbeat of embodied vitality and love."

> —**Frank Rogers, PhD**, Muriel Bernice Roberts Professor
> of Spiritual Formation and Narrative Pedagogy, and
> codirector of the Center for Engaged Compassion at
> Claremont School of Theology; and author of *Practicing
> Compassion* (named top five spirituality books in 2016
> by USA Best Book Awards)

"Those of us on a spiritual path, who have cultivated contemplative practice and engaged in social action and service of Mother Earth, are often baffled and distressed to find ourselves navigating the human condition with far less grace than we would have expected—given all the work we have done on ourselves. This book is both an explanation for and antidote to this dilemma. Alane Daugherty offers lucid, practical tools to restore sanity, soften our hearts and expand our self-compassion, and embolden us to step up as robust and joyous humans in this beautiful, broken world."

> —**Mirabai Starr**, author of *Caravan of No Despair* and
> *Wild Mercy*

"Having read Alane Daugherty's *Unstressed*, I am filled with gratitude. For she has shown me that I don't have to live with the anxiety, disease, and stress that ripple (or crash) through my daily existence. She leads me along a clear, precise path to a life of engaged compassion, a life grounded in the strength of abiding 'calm and connection.' I offer her my heartfelt thanks!"

> —**Andrew Dreitcer, PhD**, professor of spirituality, and
> codirector of the Center for Engaged Compassion at
> Claremont School of Theology

*un*stressed

How Somatic Awareness Can Transform Your Body's Stress Response and Build Emotional Resilience

ALANE K. DAUGHERTY, PhD

New Harbinger Publications, Inc.

Publisher's Note

NEW HARBINGER PUBLICATIONS is a registered trademark of New Harbinger Publications, Inc.

Distributed in Canada by Raincoast Books

Copyright © 2019 by Alane K. Daugherty
New Harbinger Publications, Inc.
5674 Shattuck Avenue
Oakland, CA 94609
www.newharbinger.com

Cover design by Amy Daniel; Acquired by Elizabeth Hollis Hansen; Edited by Gretel Hakanson

---

Library of Congress Cataloging-in-Publication Data

Names: Daugherty, Alane, author.
Title: Unstressed : how somatic awareness can transform your body's stress response and build emotional resilience / Alane K. Daugherty, PhD.
Description: Oakland, CA : New Harbinger Publications, Inc., [2019] | Includes bibliographical references. |
Identifiers: LCCN 2019017393 (print) | LCCN 2019021605 (ebook) | ISBN 9781684032846 (PDF e-book) | ISBN 9781684032853 (ePub) | ISBN 9781684032839 (pbk. : alk. paper)
Subjects: LCSH: Stress (Psychology) | Stress management. | Emotions. | Mind and body.
Classification: LCC BF575.S75 (ebook) | LCC BF575.S75 D27 2019 (print) | DDC 155.9/042--dc23
LC record available at https://lccn.loc.gov/2019017393

Printed in the United States of America

24	23	22				
10	9	8	7	6	5	4

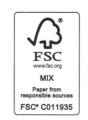
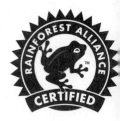

To the memory of
Kissane "Sandy" Ferguson
6/22/1927 to 11/8/2015

and

Linda Marie Rogers Kuttler
4/25/1967 to 6/11/2016

Contents

Foreword

When I was a young student at Cal Poly Pomona more than 25 years ago, I was struggling. Completely overwhelmed with the stress of academic and personal life challenges, I made some bad choices that threatened to derail my future. Fortunately, I found myself in front of Robert Naples, the dean of student affairs. With great intuition, he could see what I couldn't express: that actions aren't random, and that there were deeper reasons for the mistakes I'd made. By choosing to act from compassion instead of punition, he was instrumental in giving me the opportunity and guidance to get back on the track that led me to where I am today.

In fact, a couple of years after that incident, another seemingly small decision by someone who believed in me made a significant impact on my life. Physical education professor Ray Daugherty agreed to write a letter of reference for my application to medical school. While I'd taken Professor Daugherty's class and conducted research with him, I was amazed at the glowing praise for my character and capability that he included in his letter. I couldn't recall anyone ever believing in me that much, and his confident praise made me believe for the first time that I could really live up to those expectations.

Looking back, I've often wondered what would have happened to me if someone other than Dr. Naples had been in charge of my corrective action or if I'd not taken Professor Daugherty's class at that important crossroads in my young life. I've no idea where I might have ended up.

Today, my nonprofit organization, the Love Button Global Movement, offers a lecture series to medical students at Cal Poly and other universities through its Integrative Medicine Research and

Outreach Program. The lecture series provides the students with information on integrative medicine and whole patient care that they don't get in the classroom. It also offers support and essential information on how students can mitigate the mounting pressure and stress from highly competitive degree tracks like medicine, as well as constructive ways to maintain a balanced life outside of school. It's a healthy mix of information and intervention aimed at students who are struggling with how to manage their lives just like I was so long ago. .

So, imagine my surprise when I discovered earlier this year that the featured speaker for the inaugural lecture in the series was none other than Alane Daugherty, cofounder of the Mind and Heart Research Lab at Cal Poly—and the daughter of Professor Ray Daugherty, the professor who played a crucial role in my personal development as a young man. Her presentation was on transforming stress and anxiety into resilience and success. During her talk she shared a touching story about her father.

One morning years earlier, she was feeling particularly rushed and stressed about a certain issue as she was driving to work. Along the way, she made a conscious choice to appreciate the beauty of the mountains she was passing, a group of birds that had flown by, and even the gathering clouds. By the time she reached campus, she was calm, grounded, and fully present. At that moment, she looked up to see her father conducting a golf class in the distance. Just then, it started to pour down rain. Thinking quickly, Alane grabbed an umbrella from her car and ran it over to her father. The two of them shared a lovely moment that was simple and yet somehow profound, though Alane didn't quite know why. When there was a break in the rain, she left her father with the umbrella and hurried on to her office. Later that day, her father went home and died of a heart attack.

Had Alane not been able to neutralize her stress on that morning drive years ago, she more than likely would have been in an entirely different frame of mind when she arrived at work. She probably wouldn't even have seen her father as she trudged to her office, completely caught up in her anxiety. Instead, she chose to use the little things on her morning drive, like the beauty of her surroundings, to mitigate her stress, which resulted in a big change in her emotional state and awareness. Because of that, she now has a beautiful memory with her father just hours before his passing.

Near the end of her presentation, Alane invited my wife, Sherry, and I on stage to stress how the biggest changes in our lives are brought about by the smallest choices. When she opened the same umbrella she'd given to her dad that day in the rain over our heads, I was overwhelmed. Everything seemed to have come full circle. I was once a struggling student helped by a man who made a simple choice that made a great difference in my life. Now I was on stage at the same university with his daughter—who was helping students struggling with the same issues I had, in a program I created specifically for that purpose—under the umbrella of the man who made it all possible because he dared to believe in me.

Dr. Naples's choice to use compassion, Professor Daugherty's choice to see more in me, my choice to commit to realizing it, and Alane's choice to notice beauty—these are all simple decisions that brought about profound change at a crucial moment of decision. It's easy to become overwhelmed with the problems of life and allow stress to dictate our choices, but that can only happen if we're living unconsciously. It's easy to let stress take over and say, "This situation is too big for me. There's nothing I can do. It's out of my control," but in most cases that's not true.

Science tells us that no matter how big or complex a functioning system may be, it's the tiniest alteration within that system which holds the potential for the greatest change over time. In other words, focusing on something small and remaining consistent with it results in the biggest change of conditions. That's the power of a small change applied consistently over time. This effect is known as the law of sensitive dependence on initial conditions, or the butterfly effect.

Perhaps the greatest example of this effect was demonstrated by architect and inventor, Buckminster Fuller, who often wrote and spoke about it. I first learned about it from an article of his that was published in a 1972 issue of *Playboy* magazine that was given to me by an acquaintance. To this day, it remains the only copy of the magazine I've ever opened. Still, the article and its analogy were powerful. Fuller chose the imagery of a ship—and opted to focus on the rudder. When we see a ship's captain turn the wheel and the enormous ocean liner respond by changing direction, we assume the captain is controlling the rudder, but that's not really what's happening.

The ship's rudder is an enormous metal fan-like structure extending out and downward from the rear of the vessel like the tailfin of a fish. Because of its size, there are tens of thousands of pounds of water pressure working against the rudder, which is why it's impossible for the captain to move it with the wheel. So how does the captain do it? Running down the back edge of the main rudder is a tiny and very thin secondary rudder called a trim tab. Because it's so much smaller, it receives far less water resistance. By turning the wheel, the captain is actually controlling the trim tab; then the big rudder responds accordingly, and the ship changes direction.

There were certainly times in my life when I felt my ship was moving in the wrong direction. It was too big, moving too fast, and had too many moving parts, so I felt powerless to change any of it. Of course, that was because I was focusing on moving the whole ship instead of the tiny trim tab that would have allowed me to do so effortlessly. My trim tab was choosing to believe those who believed in me and knowing that somehow, if I did the work, all the other details would fall into place.

In *Unstressed*, Alane Daugherty provides the trim tab to this experience we call life, and the mechanism by which we can turn our ship around and set course in a new direction. The key to this process is emotional management. While we may not be able to control everything that's going on in our lives, we have total control over how we react or choose to feel about it. Changing how we feel about something changes our energy and gives us a new perspective on the situation. From a clear and conscious mindset, we can make better choices, and the ship begins to turn. Like the metaphor of the trim tab, *Unstressed* provides a path to life mastery through emotional management that's as easy to understand as it is to implement. When we learn how to manage our emotions, we have more conscious control over the quality of our lives because no matter what happens, we get to choose how we feel about it and ultimately, how we experience it. From that mindset, nothing can rock our boat as we set off for a new destination.

—Habib Sadeghi, DO
Cofounder, Be Hive of Healing Integrative Medical Center
Los Angeles
2019

Introduction

If you are like most adults, there may be a vast divide between the emotional life you long for and the emotional life you live.

You may have a deep and ever-present yearning for more. You may be longing for inner and outer calm, for connection and a feeling of wholeness. You may long to feel grounded in your own core; generatively engaged with others, yourself, and your outside world; and fully blossoming in your potential and living the life you desire. However, if you are similar to most adults, although you long to embody expansiveness and possibility, you likely experience restriction and fear because something is blocking your way.

THE PROBLEM

You may experience stress as full-blown panic or a subtle nudging that things in your life just aren't as they should be. You may experience stress as free-floating anxiety, overwhelm, worry, or fear, or it may be a result of specific circumstances in your life, such as difficulty in a relationship, fear of not being able to pay bills, or fear of not meeting yours or others' expectations. Your stress may be due to the process of life in general, the feeling that something is simply "off," or manifest as a general uneasiness, the disappointment of unmet potential, or the consequences of other untended emotional difficulties. It may be the result of how your emotional past colors your present; it may accompany a sense of helplessness or numerous other forms of self-deprecation; it may be the precursor to loneliness. It may come and go or be your constant companion. Most importantly, it may be obstructing your ability to live the life of which you are capable.

The truth is, all these things are stress. Stress blocks your ability to truly thrive, and it likely permeates your life.

As you will learn in this book, stress is, by its very definition, emotional disequilibrium. It is the experiential state of being out of emotional balance and can be caused by anything that upsets emotional balance: a thought, a word, a perception, a circumstance, a demand, a past difficult or traumatic experience, or a myriad of other things that can disrupt your emotional stability, and, consequentially, your ability to flourish. Whatever the cause, the effect is one of being knocked off balance, and it is a deeply felt emotional and experiential reality. Stress is a cyclical and escalating dance of emotional distress between your mind's perception and your all-consuming bodily response; *it is the embodied experience of emotional chaos.*

THE SOLUTION

Unstressed invites you to transform the stress in your life by transforming your emotional life. It addresses the stress in your life as an all-consuming and far-reaching problem of emotional *dis-ease*; it uses psychophysiology—how your emotional and psychological lives play out in the interconnected system of your mind and body, or your *mind-body complex*—as a platform of understanding; and it presents heartful emotion as the healing agent that transforms a life of emotional disarray to one of calm and connection. Through psychophysiology, you will see that as destructive as chaotic emotion can be, life-generating or heartful emotion may be the greatest asset you can develop. You will also see that as a "system of adaptation," you are constantly and consistently transforming to your dominant emotional experience and creating a greater capacity to live from that experience. In other words, emotional chaos begets more emotional chaos, as in stress and anxiety, but life-generating emotions, for example love, gratitude, compassion, hope, and other emotions synonymous with the heart, also beget more of the same. True and effective stress management requires reducing chaotic emotion, for sure, but then also requires actively cultivating heartful emotion as a necessary second step. Only then will you develop greater capacities to live and interpret life from the healing, hopeful, and expansive states that heartful emotion incurs.

This book is built on three underlying concepts or foundations. The first of these concepts is that you have two primary drives or systems that control your emotional life, and, from a physiological standpoint, you can only be grounded in one at a time. Each of the systems carries a very pronounced physiological imprint that causes you to see and interpret life from its dominant state. You literally perceive your current circumstance from the lens of your dominant drive. These systems are often referred to as your fear-response system, the system that is dominant when you are stressed, and your calm-and-connection system, the system that is dominant when you are feeling peaceful or relaxed. The ability to see expansiveness and possibility are primary characteristics of the latter. *Importantly, the system that you reside in most often becomes the dominant system of your life.*

These two systems were necessarily built into our species to keep us alive and flourishing: the fear response to have us automatically and immediately respond to threat, and our calm-and-connection system to encourage us to love, nurture, bond, and create community. Without either of these drives, our species would not have survived. However, given the unrelenting stresses of our current culture, your fear-response system is often in overdrive. Further, your fear response is more immediate and overpowering, with more neural connections dedicated to it, so it takes overt intentionality to cultivate your calm-and-connection system and foster its dominance. Effective stress management is a two-tiered process of reducing your fear response and actively cultivating your calm-and-connection response.

The second foundation is that emotion is the primary expression of each of these systems. When your fear-response system is in control, you are consumed with life-degenerating and destabilizing emotional responses. However, it is true, too, that when you are resting in your calm-and-connection system, you are exhibiting life-generating and stabilizing ones. The question is often posed whether emotion is "good" or "bad," and unfortunately has led to dogma that teaches us to suppress or deny all emotion. The question we should be asking isn't whether emotion in itself is good or bad, as it is often posed, but which clusters of emotion are life-generating and which are life-degenerating. We should be examining the dominant nature, quality, and context of the emotion being experienced. Simply put, as chaotic emotion is destructive and degenerating, so, too, heartful emotion is system-enhancing or life-generating.

This is consistent with the definition of emotion offered in interpersonal neurobiology by Dan Siegel, a clinical professor of psychiatry and well-known author. Siegel defines emotion as "degree of system integration" (2009). In other words, the more chaotic the emotion feels, the more it is reflected by disintegration of your neurobiological systems, or a breakdown in the coherent and optimal functioning of your mind and body, and you perceive, react, and behave from there. However, too, there are emotional states that lead to system *integration* and optimal functioning. The more you can actively engage in heartful emotion, and cultivate and reside in system-enhancing emotional states, the more you develop higher levels of neurobiological integration, and the higher capacity to live and perceive your life from those states.

Further, in his book *Biology and Emotion* (1989), Neil McNaughton, an expert in biochemistry, contends that instead of debating whether or not emotion in itself is harmful, we should take a biological approach and identify emotion by clusters. He precisely shows that different sets of emotion lead to specific and different biological and biochemical principles. Instead of looking at emotion as one general concept, he asserts, we should be identifying emotions by their impact on our overall well-being. More simply, we should identify and cultivate the clusters of emotion that lead to life generation and reduce those that do not.

The third foundation of this book is that it takes overt intentionality to cultivate what you *do* want rather than just reducing what you *don't* want; "not being sick" doesn't necessarily lead to "being well." The discipline of positive psychology demonstrates that for you to develop optimal functioning, optimal functioning needs to be the focus; and you have more agency in developing optimal functioning than you might think. This concept carries over to stress management as well. Effective and lasting stress management calls on you to not only reduce your fear response, but actively and intentionally cultivate calm and connection. In essence, it asks you to make an about-face and change your interpretation of cause and effect as it is related to your emotional life.

We often think the cause of our feelings is what's going on externally and the effect is how we feel. The cause of stress is often interpreted as the conditions of your life, and the effect is your emotional response to them. The program offered in this book invites you to reverse that understanding. In reality, the cause of your stress and anxiety is the nature and context of your emotional life, and the effect is how you interpret your external life from that lens. This book invites you to authentically and purposefully change your emotional experience and the resultant adaptations taking place, from the inside out. It invites you to actively and intentionally reduce the emotional chaos that may consume you and then transform your emotional life by engaging states that lead to flourishing and thriving. Only then can you perceive and behave differently in your presenting external life.

Basically, the program offered here uses psychophysiology as a platform for understanding that stress, anxiety, and emotional chaos are the cause of your all-consuming and presenting problem and your authentic engagement in heartful emotion is the answer to healing and transforming your emotional life. You will engage in a step-by-step process to reduce the stress, anxiety, and emotional chaos in your life by first reducing the destructive nature of your fear-response system and all its debilitating effects. You will then be invited to intentionally cultivate heartful emotion. From this cultivation, you will experience calm, connection, expansiveness, and possibility, as these are documented effects of engaging in heartful emotion and the necessary components of true thriving and well-being.

THE ROAD MAP

Unstressed is divided into three parts: understanding the problem, applying the skills, and taking it to the next level. Its unfolding is designed to guide you on your own transformative journey away from stress and emotional reactivity to calm, connection, and vitality, and to a life that's flourishing. The program offered here begins by introducing you to the scientific process of emotional transformation; then, through a step-by-step process, you are invited to experience its stress-reducing and healing capabilities in your own life. It is a progressive journey, evermore leading you from broad understanding to deep application.

Part 1 introduces you into a deeper understanding of stress and emotional disequilibrium. It also introduces you to the "spiral of becoming," a representation of how you transform emotionally from your unique perceptions, including how and why you perceive the way you do, to the meaning you attach to those perceptions, and the physiological imprint they incur—only leading to more "like" experiences. It shows you that every moment of every day, you are transforming, regardless if you are aware of it, and it can be an upward spiral or a downward spiral depending on the nature of your emotional experience. Further, it shows you the destructive capabilities of the spiral under your fear-response system. You will also be asked to reflect on how stress plays out for you in your life.

From this foundation, you will be introduced to a four-step process of recognizing, releasing, replacing, and restoring through mindful awareness and heartful engagement. You will see how these steps can lead you away from a life of stress and anxiety to one of calm and connection through emotional transformation. Lastly, you will revisit the spiral in its life-generative state when it is under the influence of your calm-and-connection system.

Part 2 walks you through the skills and deep application of recognizing, releasing, and replacing. In chapter 3, you will gain skills to subdue your fear-response system and its destructive capabilities. You will apply a specific type of mindful awareness to recognize when reactivity, stress, and anxiety are consuming your mind and body and release their hold. You will learn to recognize the dominance of your emotional attention when it is reactive and the power of a pause and present-moment awareness when it is consuming. You will learn how to tune in to your body for buried emotional truths and release harmful emotional buildup. Through this mindful recognizing and releasing, you will clear the space to effectively develop heartful engagement.

In chapters 4 and 5, you will replace reactivity with heartful engagement. Chapter 4 introduces you to heartful engagement in a general sense and walks you through specific skills to effectively cultivate it in your day-to-day life. You will learn what for you are heartful and transformative emotions, learn the power of the 3:1 ratio and intentional micromoments of connection, and develop concrete and specific ways to implement these skills in your life. Finally, you will learn the potential of affect regulation training. Affect regulation is the ability to modulate your emotional state, and it can be trained through intentional engagement in heartful emotion. HEART is a series of practices that engages heartful emotion to transform your routine affect—your embodied or experienced emotional state—leading to deep emotional transformation. Chapter 4 lays the groundwork for these and leads you through the first two foundational practices.

Chapter 5 advances your capacities for heartful engagement with prescriptions for specific emotions. It invites you to experience the significant healing potential of replacing reactivity with gratitude, self-empathy, compassion, and hope. In this chapter, you will learn the deep and healing potential of these specific emotions but also overcome the common pitfalls in their practice. You will learn the frequent mistakes people make in gratitude practice that negate its benefits and learn authentic and effective ways to practice it in your life. You will experience the deep and healing powers of self-empathy and compassion, and what it takes to cultivate true hope—not just wishful thinking. Importantly, you will deepen your affect regulation with specific HEART practices for each of these heartful emotions.

Part 3 invites you to take heartful engagement to the next level by looking at how you would most like your life to speak. In chapter 6, you are invited to look at how you can restore your capacities of resilience and flourishing. You will reflect on how you spend your time, the "stories you tell" and the "scripts you write" for yourself and others, reflect on how you interpret the events of your life, and honestly look at your deepest-held values through a meaningful examination of your life. You will practice HEART with a new and restored self-image and reflect on what you most want to bring forward into a future of restoration.

Lastly, you will be introduced to the idea that heartful engagement is an ever-deepening process. You are constantly invited to go deeper and wider with your transformation, and love is the emotion that encompasses it all. Love asks you to grow and begin to extend outward all the inner transformation you have experienced, leaving behind a life of stress and anxiety, replacing it with resilience and well-being, and spreading the transformative power of heartful emotion.

THE ESSENTIALS

Throughout this book are activities and suggestions for reflective writing that challenge you to take the journey from understanding to implementation. They encourage you to reflect and personalize the material at a much deeper level than you would by merely reading it, and completing them is an integral part of your transformational experience. Most begin as directed writing activities based on the material presented and, ultimately, invite personal reflection. The personal reflection is designed to be done in a stream-of-consciousness writing style in which you let the writing lead you. It is important to engage in the writing in this manner because reflective writing helps you put words to your emotional experience—the first step in healing it. It helps give you insight and guidance, and you are all at once better able to connect with what you intuitively know to be true about your emotional experience. We often say, "Keep the pen or pencil moving on the paper (or fingers on the keyboard) so you don't give time for the 'critic' to pop in." Just write what's on your mind and let the writing flow.

You might find it helpful to keep a personal journal dedicated to the process offered here and include thoughts or insights along your path. In addition, you might find it helpful to do the selected activities at a given time and place each day to foster consistency.

An integral part of *Unstressed* is the practice of HEART. *Heartful emotion affect regulation training* is where you most deeply experience the transformative powers of heartful emotion. The HEART practices were developed from all the scientific concepts presented in this book, and with our Western culture in mind, to be most effective and most likely practiced. There are "in-the-moment" practices designed to be done in your moments of reactivity and to transform them. There are also sustained practices intended to transform your emotional system overall. The sustained practices invite you to practice HEART for a given period of time, usually around 20 minutes, to expand and strengthen your psychophysiological experience with heartful emotion.

HEART intentionally cultivates heartful engagement often enough, and deep enough, that through routine experience, heartful emotion becomes the new "programming" from which you engage the world. Experience forms you, and experiencing HEART on a regular basis transforms your emotional system from stress and anxiety to calm, connection, resilience, and well-being. The HEART practices are an integral part of this program for transformation and should be practiced as such. All the sustained practices are available as guided audio recordings, which you can access at http://www.newharbinger.com/42839.

YOUR GUIDE

My wish for you is to not be consumed, controlled, or debilitated by the stress, anxiety, or emotional disequilibrium that surrounds you. I know that engaging from your heart heals because as a university professor, psychophysiology lab director, author, and workshop and retreat leader, I have seen it do so thousands of times. My work has offered me the opportunity to share this process of heartful engagement with thousands of people over the years. I have offered it to university students, and many other students of life, through stress-management courses, self-improvement workshops, graduate-level embodied-psychophysiology courses, retreats, and books. I have seen concrete and scientific evidence in various psychophysiology labs and have had the blessing of hearing countless personal stories of healing.

Personally, I have experienced this healing in my own life. There was a time I was so wracked with anxiety and stress, I literally couldn't function. Even though I had a master's degree in health, I had a full-blown anxiety affliction, had recurrent panic attacks, and was honestly afraid to leave the house. I was as *physically* healthy as one could possibly be, but I was falling apart from stress. I had first-hand knowledge that true and integrated health and well-being were far beyond the physical; I wanted to know what it meant to truly heal. I wanted to understand, and experience, what could transform a life from stress and anxiety to one of flourishing and vitality.

In reality, that is how this program was initially born. I genuinely dedicated my life to finding out what it meant to heal, first on a personal level, and then on academic, educational, and relational levels. After personally experiencing the deep and profound healing powers of heartful emotion, it became my life's work to share this process with those on the same journey. I went back to school, and the complete focus of my doctoral work was on healing stress and anxiety through heartful engagement. I have now been blessed to share what I have learned with multitudes of folks on the same journey.

Unstressed invites you on a scientifically based, step-by-step journey designed to transform the stress and emotional chaos in your inner and outer life by transforming your emotional life. It includes what I have learned personally, academically, and relationally from working with all the people I have been blessed to share this information with. What I have come to know through this journey is that you have it within you. Inside of you is a life of heartful engagement waiting and yearning to be born. You have within you the possibility of transformation from stress and anxiety to calm, connection, expansiveness, and possibility. You have it within you, but it takes an about-face, a change of heart, and the choice of love. It takes reprogramming some of your emotional patterning that is no longer serving you, and it takes calming the emotional chaos enough to engage heartfully and authentically with what each moment offers. Often, it takes a guide or facilitator and a blueprint for a change. This book offers you that.

part 1

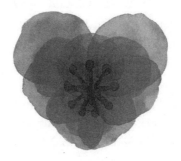

Understanding
the Problem

Part 1 lays the foundation for understanding. It introduces stress as a global and far-reaching problem in your life and, ultimately, heartful emotion as its antidote. In it, you will learn the scientific foundations of how your fear-response system runs rampant, and how, if left unchecked, it can dominate your life. It also introduces you to the healing and balancing capacities of your calm-and-connection system. It shows how a combination of mindful awareness and heartful engagement together are necessary to activate this second, more life-generating system and lays the groundwork of how to get there. This part includes both the scientific basis and an outline of your process as you journey from stress and anxiety to resilience and well-being.

It is the most content-driven and scientifically dense section of the book. It is okay to read for general understanding unless you are particularly interested in the specifics. The information shared is an important platform for the rest of the book, but don't feel like you need to retain every detail. My goal is to make it accessible for you to build a solid foundation as a basis for the rest of the program. Once this foundation has been laid, in parts 2 and 3, you will be led through a step-by-step process of implementation. Having a general understanding of the indisputable mind-body connection in emotion aids in your implementation of the science of heartfulness—your path to transforming your stress response to emotional resilience.

chapter 1

Understand Stress

Joanne would often wake up in the middle of the night with racing thoughts and free-floating anxiety. During the day, she vacillated between feeling completely overwhelmed by all her perceived demands and feeling depressed because she didn't seem to be functioning the way she wanted. She seemed to be carrying a constant sense of dread, expecting the worst at any given moment, consumed with negative self-talk, and constantly overreacting. She spent most of her time worrying about things that were likely never to happen, although in her mind, they were an imminent threat. The very lens of her existence seemed to be colored by her negative perceptions of life. Although she tried to bury her feelings and move on, the person she felt she was on the inside was decidedly different from the one she was trying to present to the outside world. She felt tired and fatigued most of the time, and the demands of her work, relationships, and responsibilities seemed too much to bear.

She longed to feel like herself once more. She longed to feel an inner peacefulness and a sense that she was truly thriving and using her gifts. She craved to be connected to her life-force—that inner radiance she knew was buried deep inside her—and fully living it in her relationships and her life. She remembered a time when she was truly happy and thought, I want to feel like that again!

Joanne longed to feel the state she knew was possible; you may have different words than she does to describe it, but you know it when you feel it. You know when your life-force is thriving, and you deeply experience it in your internal world; it is reflected in your brain, your heart, and your soul. It is what gives you the experience of being fully alive, and when you are in this state, you feel connected to both your innermost self and your outer world. Feelings of isolation, hopelessness, blame, shame, and judgment for both yourself and others disappear. You are filled with inner calm; gratitude, hope, compassion, and love are ever present in your daily life. You feel expansiveness and possibility, and you feel heartfully engaged with life itself. Whatever words you use to describe it, it is the key to healing, well-being, and higher potential. It is the life that is possible.

This state of vitality feels expanded, energetic, and free-flowing, and those qualities are decidedly absent when you aren't in this state. Unfortunately, if you are like Joanne, and most adults, you may only get an occasional whisper of this existence, if you do at all. It is likely that this effortless flow is absent from your daily life and you are immersed in stress and emotional turmoil. You may feel out of control. You may feel absent of an internal anchor. You may be living in constant reaction to the circumstances of your external life as if you have no choice in the matter. You may know there is a calmer, more expansive way to live, but you just cannot quite grasp it. Or, you may be trying to force your outer life into some semblance of fulfillment when your inner life is still in chaos and wonder why you're not happy. You may be living your life so consumed with stress and emotional chaos, loneliness, blame, shame, or judgment that you cannot even see, much less begin to live, another way. When stress permeates your days, it impacts your very interpretation of life.

And you know *that* when you feel it.

In this chapter, you will learn what stress actually is and the mechanisms that power it so you can begin to change it. You will see that as a "system of adaptation," you are constantly transforming to your life's experience through the "spiral of becoming"; a mind-body feedback loop that continually shapes your emotional life. You will see how your perceptions are unique and individual to you, molded from your life's experience. You will see that the meaning you ascribe to those perceptions forms a mind-body imprint that shapes your emotional life and alters your future perceptions. As you will discover, when under the influence of your fear-response system, this spiral can lead to a stressed-out, discontented sense of self, as Joanne experiences, or it can open you up to a sense of calm within and connection to the world—that state of inner ease and vitality that we all aspire to reach.

WHAT IS STRESS?

If I posed you the question, What is stress?, you might come up with a myriad of answers. Perhaps you would answer, as many people do, with descriptions of the *things* that stress you out: bills, family conflicts, expectations, time pressures, relationships, money issues, internal or external demands, health, and so on. You may possibly focus more on the physical manifestations of stress: too much or too little sleep, weakness, fatigue, a racing heart, headaches, gastrointestinal problems, a pit of dread in your stomach, and so forth. You might emphasize the psychological aspects: racing thoughts, forgetfulness, confusion, crying spells, overreaction, defensiveness, and so on. Or, you might concentrate on the longer-term impact of stress: depression, overwhelm, worry, anxiety, loneliness, feelings of inadequacy, hopelessness, and so forth. The truth is, stress is all these things—and not one of these things entirely.

If you look at the above lists, it may look like the things that stress you out are the causes of your stress, and your psychological and physical responses are the effects of those things. However, in reality, two people may have very different individual responses to the items on the lists. For example, one person may interpret the expectations of others as a huge stressor, and another person may have little response to those demands at all. It is really more *your personal evaluation* of the perceived threat of the items on the lists. And, as you will see shortly, your perceptions are due to your individual programming from past experience, or what you have been conditioned to recognize as threat. The things that stress you out are certainly a large part of your experience of stress, but they are not stress in and of itself.

Further, the physical and psychological turmoil you experience are more the results, or symptoms of stress, and a considerable part of your stress experience, but not the initiating factor. We can get a clearer picture of what stress actually is by looking at the initial way it was conceptualized; and, with that understanding, we can develop a better-informed plan to combat its effects.

STRESS IS EMOTIONAL AND PHYSICAL DISEQUILIBRIUM

Hans Selye was the first person to use the term "stress" as we know it today. He coined the term from mechanics, in which it was used to describe any force that disrupts the equilibrium, or free-flowing, of a machine. Humans, too, he postulated, could experience having their "free-flowing" disrupted by some internal or external force. He basically described the stress process in this way:

Your body, mind, and emotional systems want and need to be in balance. When something is perceived to be a threat, in any way, you have some sort of negative emotional reaction, and your mind-body complex responds with a cascade of negative physical reaction patterns that consume you. If the disruption is too great, lasts too long, or you repeatedly expose yourself to it, you cannot regain the balance you desperately need; you break down either physically or psychologically—or both (Chrousos, Loriaux, and Gold 1988; Hubbard and Workman 1998). And to make matters worse, through something Selye called the "general adaptation syndrome," this way of being becomes your life's primary operating pattern (Selye 1936).

What does this all mean for you? It means that stress *is* that state of emotional disequilibrium, and it can be caused by *anything* that disrupts your free-flowing state of being psychologically and physiologically grounded. It may be considerably more global and far-reaching in your life than you can imagine. It can be caused by a thought, a word, an external circumstance, or an internal feeling. *It can be caused by any disruptive emotional evaluation you bring to any circumstance.* Further, any disruptive emotional evaluation you have automatically activates your fear-response system, and, as mentioned in the introduction, when you are stressed, your fear-response system runs rampant. This causes a chaotic and tumultuous mind-body state that soon becomes your new norm.

While this all may sound disheartening and discouraging, it is actually hopeful. Understanding this process gives you a blueprint for change. When you understand what causes emotional and physical disequilibrium, in all areas of your life, and the fearful, threat-sensitive state that results, you can begin to understand how to heal it.

The first step is to dive into and deeply examine the particular disequilibrium you're feeling. That's what we'll do in the next exercise.

Exercise and Reflection:
What Is Stress for You?

The reflective writing exercises contained in this book are designed to be an invitation for you to honestly reflect on the concepts you are reading about and how they play out in your own life. You have just learned that stress can be anything that throws you off your emotional and physical equilibrium, or a balanced state of body and mind. This exercise asks for you to reflect, with a possibly new and broader interpretation of stress, on the myriad of ways stress impacts your life. Write in a stream-of-consciousness style addressing some of the following questions. The questions are not meant to be answered verbatim; they are only meant to guide your writing. Let the writing "write" you.

1. What immediately comes to mind when you think about the word "stress"?

2. What causes stress for you?

3. Are there similar situations that stress you?

4. What does it feel like generally, emotionally, and physically?

5. Are there emotional repercussions for you, such as loneliness or depression?

6. With a broader interpretation of stress, are there some things in your life you now might define as stress that you would not have before?

Brainstorm on what this thing called stress is for you, and reflect on any insights you might have gained from the writing.

Next, we will look at how you may be adapting to more of what you are experiencing now: how you are, in essence, a system of adaptation.

YOU ARE A SYSTEM OF ADAPTATION

You may be living under the pretense of a false duality. You might be operating under the assumption that your mind and body are separate—your mind either floating in space somewhere or housed solely in your brain, and your body merely the vehicle that carries you around each day. You may have been told that "you" reside in your brain and that your brain is distinctly separate from the rest of your body, or you may have been taught that your body is the part of you that is inferior, dirty, or something to transcend, a distinct liability. The discipline of psychophysiology invites you into a different paradigm.

Although most recent research in psychophysiology has been on the sub-discipline of neuroscience, or the study of the brain, in its broader context, psychophysiology shows how your emotional and psychological lives play out in all the systems of your body—and that the mind and body are indeed one, operating as an integrated whole: a mind-body complex. That is tremendously important to understand: the mind and body cannot be separated in their functioning. Any emotion you feel is experienced in your mind and felt in your body—and your bodily processes form an imprint that goes on to alter your emotional state in the future. The more emotionally driven the experience, the greater the imprint left behind. Furthermore, because you are a system of adaptation, these imprints become a template that further determines how you see, perceive, and react to your world. Basically, you are imprinted upon by what you experience, and your body-mind responds by creating a greater capacity for that experience. Every moment of every day, you are transforming to your dominant emotional experience, whether you know it or not and whether you like it or not. You are literally programming yourself to be more successful at what you routinely do.

This also means that you can manipulate what you experience to create more desired capacities. It is just like exercise or learning a math problem or how to ride a bike. Your mind-body complex responds to what it experiences, and you can create a greater capacity to live long term from any emotional state you intentionally cultivate. Unfortunately, it is usually the state of stress you live in now, but it could be that state of vitality, of fulfillment in yourself, and of heartful engagement with the world that you aspire for. The key to moving from the stressed state you are in to the heartful state you could be in is to understand *how* you adapt—to understand the spiral of becoming.

THE SPIRAL OF BECOMING

The "spiral of becoming," depicted in the following diagram, is a representation of how your psychophysiological systems of adaptation work, or, said more simply, how you are perpetually adapting or transforming. You are constantly perceiving, cultivating meaning from that perception, and registering in your body a physiological imprint consistent with the meaning you ascribe. And, as this diagram indicates, each step in the cycle of perceiving an experience, making meaning from it, and feeling the associated emotions and sensations in your body—where they remain as an imprint—influences the behaviors, reactions, and choices you make in any given moment, and they become offshoot spirals of their own!

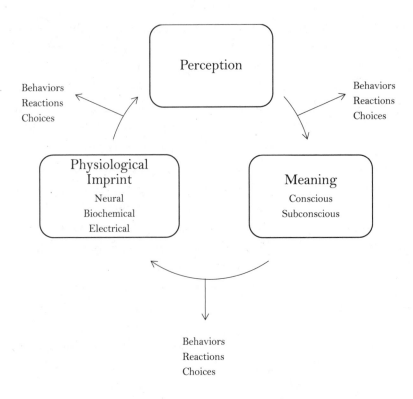

The Spiral of Becoming

Most importantly, once you embody a given imprint, you then perceive further from the lens of that imprint. It's like when you have something challenging happen in the morning, you react out of frustration,
see through the lens of that frustration, and the next event of your day
"looks" a little worse. This dynamic may go on and on until your whole
day looks like a disaster. Eighty to ninety percent of this is going on
subconsciously; you just know how you feel, think you are perceiving
the emotional truth of each circumstance, and react and transform
accordingly. This process goes on for every moment of your existence
and can be an upward spiral of favorable or life-affirming transformation or a downward spiral of adverse transformation. It all starts with
your perception, but why do you perceive things and events in your life
the way you do?

HOW THE SPIRAL WORKS: PERCEPTION, MEANING, AND PHYSIOLOGY

Every moment that you are experiencing life, you are developing perceptions based on input from both your conscious and subconscious minds. You are constantly taking in information from all your senses, both consciously and subconsciously, and this information is being sent to and filtered through the programming of the 80 to 100 billion neurons in your brain. These neurons, or nerve cells in your brain, work like "informational wiring." Alone, they do nothing, but together, these neurons form clusters, or neural nets, that connect through synapses to transfer information. These neural nets form connections based on experience, and that experience is stored as "programming" in the wiring of your brain. You may be "programmed" to be anxious in situations that have carried for you a past difficulty or to be distrustful of people that exhibit similar behaviors to someone who has hurt you before. This programming is a tangible record of experiential learning. Your brain wires to experience, and that wiring is used as a future database for all your processing. It is how all learning occurs, emotional learning included (LeDoux 1993). The larger, more impactful events of your life are embedded, or stored more strongly, as impactful experience creates more robustly connected neurons. But everything you currently experience, smell, hear, see, feel, sense, and so forth, whether you are aware or not, is processed and stored as information in the wiring of these neurons. This process is designed to provide meaning to the circumstances you are experiencing in the present, all based on what you have experienced in the past.

The way your brain attaches significance to any perception of current circumstance is to filter incoming information through its almost unfathomable memory storage of this past experience. I once had a woman in a workshop who felt transported to states of love when she smelled the combination of spaghetti sauce and cigarettes! She *felt* the response of love and security, before the conscious thought, before she even recognized why. When she was a child, she would sit at her beloved Italian grandmother's feet as her grandmother smoked and cooked. While most of us would cringe at the smell, her neural nets were coded to attach that smell with deep bonding, and her brain reacted accordingly. Further, 80 to 90 percent of this is going on sub-consciously; you just experience an emotional evaluation consistent with the processing of your subconscious brain. Because it is subconscious, you are mostly unaware, you just know how you "feel" in regard to what you are currently experiencing, never relating it to the data storage in your brain from bygone experience.

Although the spiral of becoming is proposed as a singular event, in reality, you have numerous spirals going on at any given time. You have a multitude of perceptions, both conscious and subconscious, being filtered through your system at once. You are constantly scanning everything in your environment, the obvious and the not so obvious, and evaluating according to past experience. The more significance the inner workings of your brain attaches to any present occurrence, and that occurrence could be just a thought or worry, the stronger the emotional evaluation will be. You unconsciously assign meaning to your present through the lens of your past. You know you just "feel" a certain way, most often unaware of what has contributed to that feeling or evaluation.

As you ascribe meaning or emotionally evaluate any circumstance, you immediately have physiological responses consistent with that meaning. Three main physiological systems kick in that reflect your emotional evaluation. Your neural system, or the neural networks, in your brain fire in response to the current circumstance; your endocrine system produces biochemicals consistent with how you feel in response; and your heart rate changes to reflect your emotional state, as do the electrical impulses conveyed with every beat. The greater emotional evaluation you bring to that moment, the stronger the physiological imprint. Further, the neural patterns, biochemistry, and electrical patterning, or physiological imprint of that moment, are sent back to the neural nets in your brain responsible for perception! You now perceive through that physiological imprint, and the spiral starts all over again. Also, quite importantly, at any given point in the process of that spiral, you likely exhibit behaviors and reactions or make choices consistent with the nature of the spiral. You may eat, drink, get angry, cry, or do a number of other things dependent on the nature of the spiral. Finally, the spirals you experience can travel on an upward trajectory or a downward one. It all depends on the physiological drive that's influencing them.

As you learned in the introduction, you have two primary physiological drives that compete to dominate your system at any given point in time, your fear-response drive and your calm-and-connection drive. Each drive carries its own corresponding physiological imprint. And you can't be grounded in both at once; one or the other is always dominant, and the one that is dominant most often is the one that ultimately controls your whole being. When you are stressed, your fear-response system is in control, most often in overdrive, and coloring everything you perceive, the meaning ascribed to those perceptions, and the physiological imprints they incur. The things that feel dangerous or make you vulnerable in any way—even to the level of subconscious past experience—provoke fear, anxiety, and apprehension in your body-mind: a physiological imprint of threat. As you continue experiencing stress and vulnerability, that state of threat comes on more and more frequently and comes to feel more and more natural; you begin to suffer increasingly negative effects. You begin to see the world through the lens of reactivity, and these negative effects can have significant implications for your emotional, mental and physical health; your relationships; and your life. When you're under the influence of your fear-response system, you may never realize there is another way of being.

Let's take a closer look at how the spiral of becoming plays out when it is under the influence of your fear-response system. As you read, consider how the dynamics being described might be playing out in your life.

THE SPIRAL AND YOUR FEAR-RESPONSE SYSTEM

It all starts with your individual perception. The truth is that it is not reality that drives you as much as your perception and interpretation of reality. You may think it is the person you are in conflict with, the bill you cannot pay, or your work situation that stresses you out, when in actuality it is the importance, or perception, of threat that you assign to those stressors—the way you perceive them as personally significant—that puts you on a downward stress spiral. How your brain and body perceive this personal significance—how they determine what a threat is—comes from a very primitive part of your brain that only wants to keep you safe, and that part of your brain will use any means it can to get your attention.

PERCEPTION: HOW THE AMYGDALA PERCEIVES AND REMEMBERS

Deep in your emotional brain, you have three structures—the amygdala, the hippocampus, and the anterior cingulate—that are associated with meaning-making and emotional perception. These three structures are responsible for storing and processing autobiographical memory, or memory of your personal life experience. While the hippocampus and anterior cingulate are more involved with conscious emotional memory and appraisal, the amygdala's job is to store nonconscious emotional appraisal of all your life experiences—the kind of appraisal that drives a spiral of becoming.

The amygdala is only the size and shape of an almond, but its job is enormous. Basically, it stores every experience you have ever had, filed by emotional significance, as a subconscious database to help you make meaning of your current circumstance. It is constantly scanning your environment, through all your senses, and looking for emotional matches of past experience to provide appraisal of your current circumstance. Again, this is done subconsciously, so you just perceive something to be threatening, but you are not really aware of the associations your amygdala is making.

Although the amygdala is involved in both your fear-response system and your calm-and-connection system, it is quicker and more reactive in its fear-response role, as there are more neurons dedicated to the operation of that system; you have more resources dedicated to evaluating fear and threat than calm and connection. When the amygdala evaluates threat, the reaction is immediate; and because it is subconscious, most often you are not even aware that the evaluation you are attaching to what's "in front of your face" has anything to do with your emotional past. You don't need to be; you just need to be able to identify when it is active and discern whether it is an appropriate response or not. Remember, its job is to get your immediate attention by the "whoosh" of emotional alarm.

If you have consistent triggers, or things that predictably hit your "bruised bones"—your personal ingrained sensitivities—you likely have some of your own emotional programming involved. Remember, the amygdala's job isn't to rationalize; its job is to act like a fire alarm to alert you that something in your present is sufficiently similar to something in your past that has previously hurt you or been a threat. In addition, the more emotionally laden the past experience is, the less discerning the amygdala is in matching new experiences to it. It has an inverse-response pattern: the more significant the past experience, the more generalized the current response. And it is all done beyond your conscious awareness! I once worked with a client who, as a child, had been so severely abused and traumatized by his mother that, as an adult, his amygdala fired in threat around any woman simply because of her gender.

To see how this might play out in real life, let's revisit Joanne's story.

Joanne grew up in a somewhat emotionally abusive household with a father who was both extremely demanding and emotionally unavailable. He was alcohol-dependent and often exhibited behaviors consistent with that abuse. Joanne never knew when he would explode, she always felt like she was on pins and needles, and she often took the brunt of his tirades. Joanne's mother was also unavailable on an emotional level, and because she, too, suffered from the chaos of the household, she spent a great deal of time elsewhere. Joanne felt harshly judged and largely abandoned by her parents yet felt the burden of being the caretaker of her family. Joanne was the oldest of five children in the household and was expected to care for her younger siblings because her parents did not. The expectations placed on her were unreasonably high, and she felt

like she was letting everyone down if she did not live up to them.
She was also expected to perform very well in school and was
berated badly if she struggled at all academically.

Imagine Joanne's amygdala and its emotional evaluation of her life now, as an adult. It would perceive everything to be her responsibility, and it would perceive a very real threat if she did not live up to those responsibilities. It would send terror through her system at the thought of failure and keep her on hyperalert for unexpected, undue chaos. Because her parents had rarely been there for her offering parental support, she would evaluate aloneness in having someone to lean on, understand her difficulties, or share the burdens she was carrying. Although she longed to be in a loving, trusting relationship, her amygdala would convince her that everything her partner did was either berating her or abandoning her. She would be convinced that her perceptions, what she thought was happening in a situation, were true, and her fear-response system would be in overdrive.

The truth is, we all evaluate our present life through the lens of our past experience and think we are perceiving reality just as it is. We all have emotional triggers that set off a cascade of perceptions and reactions that may be out of context for the situation. And you can often tell that it is an amygdala-driven response because the same emotional evaluation seems to play itself out in various circumstances of your life. Often, words like "always" and "never" are involved in your emotional interpretation of your life's circumstances or someone else's behavior.

Emotional triggers are your amygdala's way of saying "pay attention." The problem is, you don't hear it that way, and you assume the emotional lens you are looking through in that moment is a correct evaluation. If an emotional evaluation carries a significant mind-body reaction or it repeats often under different circumstances, chances are it is an amygdala-driven response and may be out of context for the severity of the situation. Remember, your amygdala's job is to be hyperalert in evaluating threat, but most often it is overperforming its job, and often those perceptions become ingrained patterns of reactivity, or triggers, for you.

Your job is to discern when the evaluation of threat is warranted and when a trigger drives you to respond in a way that's out of context for the situation.

Identifying your emotional triggers is a chance to identify patterns of reactivity that are amygdala-driven perceptions for you and may have become habitual ways of interpreting and responding to your environment.

Exercise and Reflection:
Identifying Emotional Triggers

This exercise asks you to reflect on things in your own life that may be emotional triggers for you. Remember, triggers are more specific than the generalized concept of stress and most often include an immediate, reactive response to something or a hyperalert evaluation of threat. The questions below will guide you to a better understanding of the situations that stress you out and the particular aspects of those situations that trigger you. You don't need to answer them in order; just use them as guides for your own exploration.

1. What are some situations, events, or conditions that you feel might be emotional triggers for you?

2. Do you have a strong response to different circumstances that have some similar components?

3. What situations do you seem to overreact to or often interpret in a threatening way?

4. What situations cause you to attach an emotional evaluation of yourself or the circumstance?

What did you learn? Did you gain any insights about how your triggers might be related to your emotional past? Use stream-of-consciousness writing to reflect in a way that is appropriate for you.

MEANING: THE STORIES YOU TELL ABOUT WHAT YOU PERCEIVE

Once you have a perception, you immediately make meaning of it. The meaning you ascribe to a given perception can be conscious or subconscious, but either way, it is your brain attaching significance to the perception to put it in the context of your present and past experience.

When meaning is made consciously, you begin to formulate a story around the perception. Again, your conscious mind senses the threat evaluation you are experiencing and wants to make sense of it in terms of your present experience. You begin to tell yourself what it means in the context of your life, right at that moment, and formulate stories about what it means from a conscious standpoint. Remember, this is all done in a split second, so it may manifest as your mind and thoughts racing, reacting as if you know the "truth" of the situation or putting it into a larger context of what someone else might mean, or their intentions, all filtered through your amygdala's often skewed interpretation of reality. It is all instantaneous, so you "just know" what you are evaluating as if it were the only possible understanding of reality. You match the "whoosh" of feelings you are experiencing with what is present in your awareness and begin to validate your experience.

Because your amygdala's job is to constantly scan your environment and release threat perceptions consistent with what it perceives, if and when they reach conscious awareness, your thoughts and inner chatter may run rampant. It is estimated that you have between sixty and eighty thousand thoughts a day, 80 percent of those thoughts are repetitive, and at least 80 percent are negative. An overactive amygdala prompts your conscious mind to release those thoughts with a vengeance. Your conscious mind, then, may catastrophize, telling you every catastrophe it can dream of. It may play conversations or dire scenarios in your head. It may tell you the worst versions of reality it can think of and get you to believe them. It seems you cannot shut your mind up when it is in this form of overdrive. It is relentless in its constant chatter. Worse, your brain doesn't know the difference between something that is vividly imagined and reality, so you actually begin to cultivate a greater capacity for believing and creating those scenarios. The structures in your brain, under the influence of your fear-response system, are incessant talkers, powerful storytellers, and deafening doomsday predictors.

Exercise and Reflection: Inner Chatter

Process and reflect on the endless reels of inner chatter you play all day, every day. Write in a stream-of-consciousness style addressing some of the following questions. Remember, the questions are not meant to be answered verbatim; they are only meant to guide your writing.

1. What thoughts tend to consume you?

2. What do you tell yourself about yourself or the circumstances you experience?

3. What stories do you tell yourself as you perceive your moment-to-moment existence?

4. Do you catastrophize, and, if so, about what?

5. What dire interpretations and meanings do you bring to your daily situations and involvements?

What did you learn about your inner chatter? Can you make a connection between the nature of your inner chatter and the way your amygdala works? Process and reflect in a way that is appropriate for you.

Besides the conscious meaning you assign to your various perceptions, you also ascribe subconscious meaning to them. In fact, somewhere around 80 to 85 percent of your perceptions and resultant meanings remain subconscious. How would the meaning you assign to a perception be subconscious?

A good example is the time I got that phone call that every parent is terrified to get. My son had fallen into a window, and the glass severed a central part of his arm, including a major artery. He was in grave danger of bleeding to death very soon; they were putting him on a helicopter to airlift him to a trauma unit to hopefully save his life. Obviously, a traumatic event for both of us, one that my amygdala made sure to imprint quite solidly in my brain. Although he made it through the six-hour surgery, and even kept his arm, for months after, I had major stress reactions every time I heard a helicopter. I would feel extreme anxiety before I was even consciously aware that I was hearing a helicopter. I would be walking across campus, and it would hit: I would have trouble breathing; my heart would race; I would feel embodied alarm and not know why. I would stop and pause to try and figure out what was going on, and *then* I would hear the helicopter.

Unbeknownst to me, my subconscious perception was filtering my environment, hearing the helicopter, ascribing to it the meaning of threat, and sending out an all-consuming physical-alert response. It was all beyond my conscious awareness until I felt the anxiety. The initial perception was subconscious, the meaning my amygdala made of hearing the helicopter was subconscious, but the physical reaction I felt was overwhelming.

While it is clear why my amygdala perceived the helicopter to be an extreme threat—because of the association with my son's accident and the imprint that experience left behind—it was way off base in considering the helicopter itself a threat. Remember, the amygdala's job isn't to rationalize; it is to react. It reacts before one has time to think and from how it has been programmed, whether the reaction makes any sense or not. And it does its job amazingly well.

What also do their jobs well are the neural, biochemical, and electrical systems that kick in, as the amygdala does, to create imprints like the one that the helicopter activated for me. Let's look at those next.

THE PHYSIOLOGICAL IMPRINT: WHEN THREAT BECOMES EMBODIED

Once you perceive and make meaning of a perception, again within or beyond conscious awareness, you immediately respond with a physiological imprint, or an embodied response of the emotional evaluation you attach to that meaning. In other words, you simply embody how you feel about what you are perceiving. This happens throughout your whole mind-body complex; the three systems heavily interact and influence one another in the physiological imprint they incur, and they further develop your emotional capacities in the current direction of your "spiral of becoming." Your neural, biochemical, and electrical systems deeply transform to and reflect your state of fear response, creating long-term adaptations that increase your capacity to live from these states.

The science behind how these three systems interact and reflect your emotional experience can be quite dense. My goal is to not lose you in the details, but to make the science accessible and give you enough foundational information to see how stress negatively affects both your momentary functioning and your long-term adaptations. It is from this understanding that you will see how detrimental remaining in stressed states and emotional chaos is to your life unless you replace them with more life-generating emotional experiences. We will start with revisiting neural imprints.

Neural Imprints

Your neural systems are not only responsible for original perceptions; they are responsible for perpetuating those perceptions and continuing your fear-response story unless you give them different experience. We will recap just a bit to help you put neural activity in the context of how you continually adapt.

Your neural nets are clusters of neurons that serve as the wiring of your nervous system, specifically in your brain. They wire to any experience you have and serve as "programming" for your brain to interpret and make sense of new events. The way they connect is through synapses between single neurons that reflect and then record your experience; experience is then filed according to emotional significance. What's more, your neurons record the original experience, as you learned in the discussion of perception, and they also record *repeated evaluations around those perceptions*, including words, thoughts, and any other behaviors or reactions. For example, if you struggled taking a test in the past and that experience caused you to be nervous every time you faced a new test, those particular neural nets would repeatedly fire; you could eventually create full-blown test anxiety just by your response patterns.

Joseph LeDoux (2002), one of the original researchers of the fear-response system and neural activity, says it simply: "You are your synapses" (ix). Your synapses reflect your continued thought processes, evaluations, and the way you perpetuate your perceptions, and you further adapt to their pattering of firing. Further, around the synapses are glial cells that function somewhat like glue. The more you have any repeated experience, and it could be just perceiving or responding to an event or circumstance the way you always have, the more the glial cells help facilitate long-term connections. This makes them stronger and more efficient for repeated patterns. Thus, neurally, you become better at the things you routinely do: the experiences you have, the behaviors you exhibit, the thoughts you think, and the emotions that surround all those things. When your neural nets are constantly firing under your fear-response system, you are training that system to be in control of your life. You perpetuate that reality unless you offer them a different experience or a new pattern of firing.

It is important to understand that when your fear-response system is in control, acting, reacting, and perceiving the way you always have just cultivates the capacity for more of the same. If I had continued to react with heightened anxiety every time I heard a helicopter, I would have just cemented those reactions in my neural nets. I could have developed even worse anxiety around the event itself, and that anxiety would likely have extended to issues around my children's health as a whole; generalizing in that nature is an inherent function of your stress response.

Biochemical Imprints

In addition to your neural system, your biochemical system plays a significant role in your spiral of becoming and profoundly effects how you feel at any given point in time. Biochemicals are simply chemicals that travel throughout your whole body and have a specific job to do; they work in conjunction with receptor sites. Every cell and organ in your body has receptor sites for various biochemicals. Receptor sites are molecules responsible for receiving the chemical messages and causing some form of cellular response. Together, their influence is enormous. There is not a cell in your body that is beyond the influence of your biochemistry, and the biochemicals of emotion are especially powerful.

When your biochemical system is active under your fear-response system, it floods your body and brain with chemicals, like adrenalin and cortisol. These biochemicals help you react in times of danger, cause a hyperalert response in you, *and* increase your capacity for more long-term stress, predisposing you to feel more of it, more often.

When your amygdala determines a threat, it automatically and immediately sends that message of threat to your hypothalamus, pituitary, and adrenal glands—what's called your HPA axis, which serves as a biochemical production plant for the stress hormones that go on to flood your body. First, your hypothalamus, located in your brain, produces a hormone called corticotropin-releasing factor, or CRF, that triggers your pituitary, also in your brain, to generate adrenocorticotropic hormone, or ACTH. ACTH travels to your adrenal glands, which sit in the small of your back on top of your kidneys, and stimulates them to release the primary stress hormones, adrenalin and cortisol. Basically, the important point here is that when your brain perceives threat, it launches a multistage process to flood your whole body with stress hormones.

Adrenalin, or epinephrine, is a fairly quick-acting hormone, meant to help you react to an immediate threat. It works quickly, raising your heart rate and blood pressure, but it also dissipates fairly quickly, allowing you and your body to recover. However, cortisol is much longer lasting, more complex, and much more damaging.

Cortisol, in and of itself, is not bad; you need a certain amount of it to function optimally, even to get out of bed in the morning. In its balanced state, it helps control your blood sugar, regulate your metabolism, and reduce inflammation. It keeps you focused and alert for long periods of time. Unfortunately, you likely have far too much of it because of the nature of the stress you experience and its unrelenting effects.

Cortisol is related to a whole host of physical and mental side effects. The physical effects include diabetes, increased inflammation, increased body fat, increased heart disease, premature aging, a suppressed immune system, gastrointestinal system problems, lower life expectancy, early death, and the list goes on. Mental effects include a myriad of stress-related disorders including depression, anxiety, loneliness (Doane and Adam 2010), decreased resilience, memory and learning issues, and increased mental illness. It also causes cortical inhibition, meaning you cannot recall stored information, like not being able to recall what you know when taking a test or being able to remember your phone number when you are in a car accident.

Too much cortisol can be devastating for your mental and physical health—especially since cortisol is a long-acting hormone. It has a twelve-hour half-life—meaning that, twelve hours after cortisol first floods your system, it only takes half as much additional cortisol to get you back to the original level of the primary upset. In other words, it stays in the body at fairly high levels for long periods of time. Further, cortisol receptors can be found in almost all the cells in your body (Guyre and Munck 1998).

Besides the devastating effects that too much cortisol can have on your general health and momentary responses, some very harmful adaptations take place in your fear-response system if all stress hormone levels are too high, for too long. First, if your ACTH levels are elevated for too long, it prompts your adrenal glands to make more adrenocorticotropic cells—the cells that actually produce cortisol. Basically, your body thinks it needs more cortisol to keep up with the threat response it is receiving, so you just make more cortisol-producing cells. Further, when your cortisol levels then are higher, you upregulate receptor sites in cortisol-receiving cells, allowing them to take in more cortisol. Sometimes, these cortisol-saturated cells can even change the way a gene is expressed.

Although science used to state that your genetic makeup predetermined certain aspects of your existence—that genes alone controlled your biology—we are now learning differently. Epigenetics is an area of science that shows how certain genes can be activated or deactivated by the biochemicals they are exposed to. That is, the DNA itself is not changed, but the way the gene expresses itself is. Simply put, your biochemical makeup can actually change the way a gene functions, and the biochemicals of emotion are particularly impactful this way. High levels of cortisol have been shown to change the expression of a gene associated with depression and anxiety called SERT 5HTT.

SERT 5HTT is a serotonin transporter gene. People have different forms of this gene; one specific form was identified as a contributing factor in stress, depression, and anxiety disorders. It was an important finding but disheartening for those who had this genetic characteristic. Did that mean they were doomed to experience anxiety or depression?

A series of very important studies found that it wasn't necessarily the genetic tendency that caused these disorders, but the external influences that enabled the genetic tendency to be expressed. Specifically, it was the level of cortisol people were exposed to that determined whether the gene would be "activated" and anxiety or depression would develop. Put another way, the specific form of the gene wasn't as problematic as the amount of cortisol it was exposed to, and that was due to the level of stress response a person experienced. Furthermore, it wasn't a single large surge of cortisol that changed the gene's expression so much as "low grade" cortisol baths—steady streams of cortisol experienced all day long, primarily due to thought processes surrounding emotional issues. For example, these streams might be caused by the endless loops of negative things you say to yourself, the harmful conversations you have in your head, and the way you might replay negative events instead of healing them. These low-grade cortisol baths can be as damaging or even worse than the events that precipitate them because you are exposing yourself to a steady influx of cortisol all day.

To review, when your stress response is activated more than is healthy for you, you respond biochemically by producing excess amounts of cortisol, which can profoundly impact your overall health and how you feel, think, and respond; it also causes your brain and body to go into high alert. Almost every cell in your body is affected, and you undergo long-term adaptations that just further your stress capabilities. These adaptations include making more cortisol-producing cells, making more receptor sites in the cells to absorb more cortisol, and possibly even altering a genetic tendency toward anxiety and depression. Your biochemical responses are deeply connected back to your thoughts and emotions by a feedback loop and continue this destructive process unless you change your emotional experience. The good news is, you can deliberately reduce your stress response and cultivate balance by working with the underlying thoughts, perceptions, and emotions that drive your system.

Biochemical influences are also connected to the electrical patterning of your heart. We'll look at that next.

Electrical Imprints

Your heart is an amazing organ. Although it is quite often thought of as a mere pump, it is more intricately connected to your emotional-response systems—your fear-response system and your calm-and-connection system—than you might think. Your heart is in constant two-way dialogue with your brain in a feedback loop of emotional evaluation and response. It receives information regarding your emotional state from your brain, for sure, but it also has its own inherent system of emotional reflection that, in turn, gets sent back to some very important parts of your brain, and is detected throughout your body. The way this happens is through electrical patterning.

What allows your heart to beat and send biochemicals, oxygen, and nutrients to all the cells of your body is the electrical impulse that stimulates it. Your heart is largely hollow and comprises cardiac muscle tissue on the outside; the electrical impulse causes this muscle tissue to contract and force the blood within it throughout your body. It actually speeds up and slows down with every beat because it is constantly responding to your emotional and physical needs. The electrical impulse is intrinsic to the heart itself, meaning that your heart doesn't depend on your brain for the impulse to beat. You have a small mechanism in the top right section of your heart called a sinoatrial node, or SA node, that provides that electrical impulse. That is why someone, after a serious accident, can be "brain-dead" in the hospital yet still have a beating heart. In essence, the heart has its own intrinsic nervous system.

In addition, within your heart's nervous system are various receptors: mechanisms responsible for picking up physiological cues from your body regarding its chemical state and pressure state. Some researchers additionally believe it has its own system of perception and type of memory (McCraty 2015). Upon receiving these clues, the SA node sends out electrical impulses consistent with the quality and context of those clues, and the heart beats accordingly. It is kind of like the Morse code of the body. This is what causes your heart to speed up and slow down with every beat, and its variability patterns can reveal a lot about your emotional state.

Heart rate variability is a measurement of beat-to-beat time changes in heart rate. When it speeds up and slows down in a consistent and smooth pattern, the impulses are likely reflecting a calm and balanced emotional state; the "Morse code" signals the SA node sends out are ones of calm. When the electrical impulses are speeding up and slowing down in a chaotic pattern, they are likely reflecting an emotional state full of disequilibrium—or stress and anxiety—and the heart sends out that corresponding "Morse code." Researchers use the term "heart coherence" to define the continuum of the smoothness of the state; high coherence reflects a very smooth pattern of heart rate variability, and incoherence has a very jagged or inconsistent pattern.

It is like your heart is a detection-and-magnification system that takes physiological information about your emotional state, puts it into a code of electrical patterning, and sends it throughout your body. One of the most significant places this patterning is sent is back to the brain by way of the vagus nerve. It is sent to both your prefrontal cortex—a part of your brain wanting to consciously evaluate your emotional experience—and back to your amygdala, which senses the patterning, reacts, and continues the feedback loop of threat and alarm unless the patterning is changed. Both of these brain areas contribute to your continued conscious and subconscious stress response patterns until your emotional experience changes.

Simply put, when activated, your heart transmits chaotic electrical impulses that carry messages throughout your body by the way they are patterned. Your body, being a phenomenal pattern detection system, picks up these patterns throughout, especially in some very important and influential parts of your brain. These parts of your brain send an immediate message back to your body to release a flood of chemicals that tell you how to feel, how to react, and how to guide your further perceptions—which repeats the spiral all over again!

As you will see throughout the rest of this book, there are things you can do to intentionally engage and shift your level of heart coherence, the way you perceive and perpetuate stress and threat, and profoundly change your emotional resilience, outlook, and ability to engage with your life. But first, let us look at how a fear-driven response system may manifest for you. The easiest way to figure out what your fear-response spiral—and the physiological imprint it leaves behind—looks like for you is by reflecting on how it feels as you experience it.

Exercise and Reflection: Your Personal Physiological Imprint

Your fear-response drive carries a pronounced physiological imprint. Process and reflect on the myriad of ways you may physically express your fear-response drive and what you think your physically reactive patterns are. Remember, because a fair amount of your fear response may be beyond conscious awareness, noticing the way it manifests in your body is a great tool to recognize when it has become active. Tune in to your body and reflect on the following questions, answering them in a stream-of-consciousness style. Remember, the questions are not meant to be answered verbatim, they are only meant to guide your writing.

1. What do you think your physical patterns of reactivity are?

2. How can you remind yourself to tune in and be present to their messages?

3. Where in your body are your physical patterns of reactivity most present?

4. Do you always feel them in specific patterns of response, or do different situations carry different responses? If so, what are they?

5. How can you learn from these physical cues to identify what your physical patterns of reactivity root causes are, or what may be activating you?

Process and reflect in a way that is appropriate for you. Also consider how you can take the knowledge you gained from this activity and implement it in your life.

When we look at the spiral of becoming, it is a little like trying to figure out which came first, the chicken or the egg. In other words, it is an ongoing cycle or spiral, and there really is no beginning or end. The whole process is continually perpetuating itself. Your neural system, biochemical system, and electrical system work in concert in reflecting any emotional state you are currently experiencing, and they also adapt in their own specific ways to cultivate more of the same. This means that you are constantly becoming more of any emotional state you are consistently experiencing—and you are seeing your world from that state. In addition, this all goes back to how your personal and individual perceptions were created in the first place.

Let us revisit Joanne's story and look at how this played out for her.

Because of her past, the amygdala-driven perceptions of her present and the meaning she ascribed to them, Joanne's stress response was constantly in overdrive. She always thought people were judging her for not being good enough, and her work-life suffered. In her personal life she felt physically overwhelmed with her perceived responsibilities, and although she longed to be in a loving relationship, she was on high alert every time her partner did anything that threatened her or reminded her of her father. It could be more overt, like a similar situation, or as simple as a facial expression, attitude, gesture, or smell. Regardless of whether she was aware of the trigger or not, she would experience an anxiety-filled reaction with an all-consuming physical response. Her mind would race, her heart would race, and she would feel completely overwhelmed and often unable to catch her breath. She would tell herself stories to validate her physical experience of threat and begin to believe those stories. She couldn't calm the emotional chaos enough to see any situation clearly, and she assumed her current circumstances warranted the strength of her emotional and physical response. The anxiety she felt was all-consuming, and although she hated feeling like that, it began to be her familiar state of being. She was reacting as if today were yesterday, and her adaptive systems kicked in and began to be the lens through which she saw the world. Her continuing behavior and attention furthered the cycle. Every thought, her choice of words, "loops" of inner chatter, and her big response patterns as well as smaller response patterns continued her downward spiral. She knew there had to be a better way.

As Joanne's story shows, "stress" is, again, a state of emotional and physical disequilibrium—basically, anything that throws you off balance, emotionally and physically—that is intimately related to other difficult emotional states such as loneliness, hopelessness, depression, and anxiety; and it is all-encompassing and *embodied*. You feel its debilitating effects. And the more deeply embodied or "felt" a given experience of stress is, the greater the physiological imprint it leaves behind.

In Joanne's story, we also see the psychophysiological insight that you are a "system of adaptation," constantly reflecting and molding, emotionally and physiologically, to any experience you have. You see the world through the lens of your own unique perception and react accordingly, and this forms an experiential blueprint that continues to shape your perceptions of, reactions to, and embodiment of future experience. In other words, the experiences you have transform you, creating greater capacities for more of the same. As such, the way to heal the stress, emotional chaos, and anxiety that consume you is to offer yourself a different, more life-generating experience. Effective stress management and true healing are not just about stopping what is wrong, they are about intentionally creating what is right.

And, if you are where Joanne is, this insight can give you hope.

CONCLUSION: THERE IS HOPE

As you learned in the introduction to this book, you have two primary physiological systems that dictate, respond to, and further guide your emotional life. These are your fear-response system and your calm-and-connection system. In this chapter, you saw the downward and destructive capabilities of the spiral of becoming—the spiral formed by the interplay between your perception of the world, the meaning you make of it, and the physiological imprint that results—when you are under the influence of your fear-response system. The good news is that with intentionality, understanding, and application, you can replace the downward spiral of your fear-response system with the upward spiral of your calm-and-connection system. With new experience, you rewire implicit memory, change your perceptions, attach different conscious and subconscious meanings to those memories, and foster positive physiological imprints. Doing so short-circuits your stress response. Your neural patterning improves, your biochemistry shifts, and the electrical patterning of your heart becomes more coherent. These shifts change the nature of the spiral altogether, and you reverse your cycles of adaptation from stress and anxiety to calm and connection.

In the next chapter, you will gain an understanding of the mechanisms of change and be introduced to a blueprint of implementation built on the scientific concepts you learned in this chapter. You will learn how emotion can be destructive or constructive and how the nature of it reflects the degree of your whole psychophysiological, or embodied, system integration. You will be introduced to a process designed to first reduce the impact of your fear-response system, through a specific application of mindful awareness, and then to intentionally cultivate your calm-and-connection system through heartful engagement. By recognizing, releasing, replacing, and restoring, you will learn how your spiral of becoming transforms to a spiral of calm and connection and leads you on the path from stress and anxiety to emotional resilience and flourishing.

chapter 2

Integrate Emotion

*It was a challenging morning getting the kids off to school, and
I was pressed to make it to work on time. Everything that could
go wrong was going that way. It was raining, and there was major
construction both near my house and at the university where I
teach. My mind was racing with all the exaggerated and negative
interpretations I was bringing to the morning: what a horrible
mother and professor I was, all the awful things that could happen
if I were five minutes late, how I just couldn't "get it together," and
so forth. As my mind raced, my body reacted, and I could feel my
anxiety level skyrocketing. I had just enough time to make it if there
were no hitches. The stress was building, and I could feel its impact.
Immediately I was delayed, and I was beginning to feel the stress of
time, furthering the frustration of the morning. "I'm still okay,"
I thought. There was a faculty parking lot right next to the building
I taught in, and I could always find a parking spot there.*

*That is, until that morning. I was shocked and dumbfounded
when there were no spaces. I had to drive all the way around to
another lot where I would have to cross several muddy grass athletic
fields, a long walk in the rain carrying numerous bags for my heavy
teaching load. Beyond stressed and anxious, my inner chatter
intensified, telling me how dire the situation was and relating all the
upsetting things that were surely to come of it.*

*As I began to make my way, with all my bags, through the mud
and the rain, miraculously, some voice deep within me cut through*

all the negative chatter and reminded me: "Bring yourself present,
Alane. Look for the opportunity."

Something incredible happens when you bring yourself truly
present. For me, the shift was palpable, and, given the emotional
state I was starting from, what happened in the next several minutes
was nothing short of amazing. Immediately I began to feel the soft
rain on my face and appreciate its texture. For the first time, I saw
the loveliness of the morning. The fields were actually beautiful, and
behind them, I could see the snow-topped mountains. As I noticed
these things, my "brain chatter" and the overexaggerated emotional
significance I was bringing to the morning began to quiet. I felt a
measurable shift in both my physical and emotional state, and, for
the first time since I woke, my laser focus of stress dissipated, and
I began to let in the expansive beauty of life. I even found some
amusement in the mishaps of the morning. That shift made me
much more available to the opportunity of the moment, and that
moment offered something surprising.

· I ran into my dad. We both taught for the same department at
the university, but because I always came in from the other side,
I almost never saw him. He was teaching a golf class, on the grass
fields, in the rain. I had no idea he had a class in that space or at
that time. I cannot explain exactly what happened at the instant
that I saw him; all I can say is that sometimes life intervenes, makes
magic, and offers heart-to-heart connections with another that are
impossible to put into words. This was one of them.

Although I was peripherally aware that my class was still
waiting, being fully present in this moment with my father seemed
more important. I dropped all my bags and playfully held the
umbrella for him as if he were a king and the most important person
in the world. I will never forget that moment of genuine eye contact,
full presence, and heart-to-heart engagement. He laughed.
I laughed. His class laughed. The rain became a downpour,
and he excused his golfers for drier conditions.

I entered the building, and while I was walking down the
hallway to meet my class, I reflected on what a transformational

moment that had been. Even though I was wet and muddy and a few more minutes later to my class than I would have been otherwise, what I was bringing to my class in the way of my emotional presence was night and day. Instead of coming in to my class frazzled, harried, stressed out, and emotionally unavailable, I came in fully present, full of love, and ready to connect with my students.

I had experienced a tangible reminder of the importance of presence, and if the story had ended there, it would have been enough.

It didn't.

I went on to teach my class, full of the love and connection that had been exchanged between my dad and me, and I somehow knew that was a significant moment for us. But my dad had another story. After he canceled his class, he started not feeling well. He decided to leave work for the day and go home to rest. While at home, he had a massive heart attack and passed away. That was the last time I ever saw or spoke with him.

I have thought of that story many times since and the absolute grace I was given to hear that deep voice within reminding me to be present in the moment and look for the heartful opportunity. I can only imagine how different the story would have been if my last words to him had been: "Dad, I cannot talk right now. It has been a horrible morning, I am stressed out, and I am late for class. I am sorry, I just do not have the time."

As you know, you have two distinct ways of being in the world: the all-consuming, chaotic state of your fear-response system and the state of being rooted in your calm-and-connection system, an expansive, grounded sense of union with yourself and everything around you. As you learned in the introduction, this is consistent with the definition of emotion as "degree of system integration." As chaotic and destructive as some emotional states can be, others can be life-generating and "system-integrating." These are the states where you are grounded in your mind and body and functioning at your emotional and physical best. To most effectively reduce the stress and anxiety in your life and replace it with resilience and flourishing, both ends of the "integration continuum" must be addressed.

That morning with my father, I experienced both, and being able to shift from one to the other is a moment I will always be grateful for. Two things needed to happen to make that moment a possibility. I needed to be able to subdue the emotional chaos that was consuming me, and then I needed to be able to authentically engage with the possibilities before me.

Mindful awareness allows you to achieve the first of these steps; heartful engagement permits the second.

Mindful awareness quiets an out-of-control fear-response system, a necessary first step in being able to shift the system that is dominating your awareness, and heartful engagement intentionally fosters a calm-and-connection system. In this chapter, you will learn the power of emotion in the context of both spirals. You will learn just how mindful awareness and heartful engagement can be brought together to change your emotional experience and activate your calm-and-connection system. This turns the downward spiral of becoming you experience under your fear-response to an upward one. You will be introduced to the process of recognizing, releasing, replacing, and restoring, and you'll see just what your mind-body complex looks like when you're in a calm and connected state.

First, you are invited into an exercise and self-reflection. This exercise is dedicated to the experiential understanding of your two physiological systems, as experiencing them from an embodied state gives you a deeper grasp on their power. Your engagement in the following exercise will provide a richer understanding of how these two drives profoundly affect how you feel, psychologically and physically, how you interpret the world from these states, and the power of your focused attention.

Exercise and Reflection: The Feeling States of Awareness

Part 1. Vividly write about an event or time period where you felt particularly stressed. It does not have to be the most severe time in your life, although it can be if that is what you choose. It can be a smaller stressful event that happened recently. The key is to choose a time where you really felt stress and the associated emotional upheaval and to describe, with time and thought, the event that caused it, in as much detail as possible. Include responses to the following prompts:

1. Describe the event or time period.

2. Detail how you felt generally or psychologically (such as overwhelmed, tired, anxious).

3. Detail any specific physical sensations you felt (for example, headache, racing heart, pit in stomach).

4. Describe how you physically feel right now, recalling the event (not how you felt in retrospect).

Part 2. Now write about a time where you felt particularly happy, "in the zone," or grounded in your essence. Again, this does not have to be the most impactful time of your life, although it can be if you choose it to be. It just has to be a time when you truly felt the sensations of happiness or coherence in yourself and the situation. Write within the exact same guidelines as described above.

1. Describe the event or time period.

2. Detail how you felt generally or psychologically.

3. Detail any specific physical sensations you felt.

4. Describe how you physically feel right now, recalling the event (not how you felt in retrospect).

Part 3. Reflect, summarize, and process the exercise, the questions, and what resonated with you most throughout this experience. Write in a stream-of-consciousness style. Remember, the questions are not meant to be answered verbatim; they are intended to guide your thinking.

1. What was this whole experience like for you?

2. How easy was it for you to think of something to write about, and how enthusiastically did you begin writing during each event?

3. Did you reexperience the same feelings as you relived the events?

What was this exercise like for you? Consider the physiological and psychological states that accompanied your experience. If you were able to deeply engage in the exercise, you likely recalled events that, for you, carried very different ways of experiencing life. In the writing about a stressful event, you likely recalled a time when your fear-response was in control and dictating your perceptions and interpretations and you were feeling its effects. You likely felt some physical and psychological effects that were deeply intertwined, creating a whole mind-body response to the situation you were experiencing. You may have even reexperienced those states as you were writing about them. This exercise is helpful in allowing you to recall the experiential aspect of your fear-response system. It is a deeply embodied, physically felt state of being.

It may have been harder for you to allow yourself to focus on a happy time. However, if you were able to really focus on such a time, you likely felt a shift. You may have been able to recall the mind-body state associated with that time, and it was likely very different from the first experience. You may have felt more expansive; you may have felt lighter. You may have even smiled a bit when you were writing and experienced those states again.

This exercise hopefully gave you an experiential lesson of your fear-response and calm-and-connection systems. While the stressful situation was probably a good representation of your fear-response system in action, the happy or joyful event was likely one of your calm-and-connection system. You may have been able to feel the difference.

But how do you learn to reduce the harmful effects of one while cultivating the beneficial effects of the other? Looking at emotion as "degree of system integration" provides the answer.

UNDERSTAND EMOTION AS SYSTEM INTEGRATION

When you look at emotion in the context of physiological system integration, you can readily see that when you are in states of emotional upheaval, your whole system is disrupted and you see, react, and behave from those states. You can also see that there are emotional states that allow a sense of full presence, connection, and groundedness. You may have experienced these states as you were doing the previous exercise. The way to move up the continuum of system integration is to actively diffuse your fear-response so you can intentionally engage your calm-and-connection system.

Let us go back to the morning with my father. As the stress of the morning intensified, my whole mind-body complex began to react with a fully embodied state of stress and anxiety. Making things much, much worse, the more I succumbed to the crazy anxiety I was feeling, the worse was my exaggerated evaluation of the situation. Both my mind and my body were in high threat, and the more attention I gave to it, the worse it got. If I had run into my father before I took the chance to intentionally counteract the fear-response that was consuming me, I would have never been available to engage with him the way I did. It was the dual emphasis of quietening my internal chaos and then intentionally connecting to the available love in my presence that allowed that moment to evolve. I paused, I became present, and *then* I engaged, moving myself up the continuum of system integration. And that's how you break out of fear-response states and enter calm-and-connected ones.

When your fear-response system is running rampant, it is in control, and without first diffusing its all-consuming power, your calm-and-connection system is elusive at best. So, effective stress management requires you to both stop your habitual response patterns to stress and reactivity, quietening your internal chaos, and then create new and restorative ones. The concepts of mindfulness and heartfulness are like two halves of a transformative and healing whole; combined, they give you the necessary elements to reduce the stress and anxiety that consume you and cultivate a calmer and more connected existence.

APPLY MINDFUL AWARENESS TO SUBDUE YOUR FEAR RESPONSE

Mindfulness, or mindful awareness, is most often described as a full presence of mind, from a nonreactive, nonjudgmental, fully accepting posture. It basically means that you are using your conscious attention to be mindful of both your internal and external circumstances without engaging in reaction, judgment, or emotional interpretation about them. Sometimes it is described as "cultivating the witness," or "becoming the observer" of your own impulses, the impulses of others, and your outside environment—maybe even doing so with a little curiosity. In its purest sense, it is void of the reactivity that so often consumes your moments; hence it is the necessary foundation to calming an activated fear-response system. When you can observe your response but disengage from the need to react, you can more easily maintain a grounded way of being. This, then, begins to open space to reshape all your typical and preprogrammed response patterns.

The cultivation of mindful awareness calms your fear-response drive and rewires your ingrained reactive patterns. Through a nonjudgmental disengagement from the reactivity of your fear response, mindful awareness subdues the spiral from spinning out of control. Practicing mindfulness helps you not succumb to the chaotic inner chatter of an overactive amygdala and lessens the catastrophic meaning you typically attach to circumstance. It breaks the neural connections of your typical response patterns and begins to reduce your cortisol and smooth the electrical patterns of your heart. All this causes foundational changes in your perceptions, your behaviors, and your ability to be grounded in the present moment, which further fosters nonreactive and accepting ways of being in the world. It allows you the gift of full presence, but it is only the beginning.

APPLY HEARTFUL ENGAGEMENT TO CULTIVATE CALM AND CONNECTION

A heartfully engaged approach to stress and emotional chaos invites you to not only reduce your fear response and the harmful effects of that state, but to intentionally and actively cultivate a contradicting one. It is not just about reducing what is wrong; it is about intentionally creating what is right.

Heartful engagement is about the active cultivation of life-generating emotional states, which allow your calm-and-connection system to dominate. When you look at what defines "life-generating" through the science of embodiment, you can clearly see that there are specific states of being that lead to a dominant calm-and-connection system and that nurture life, and there are those that do not. As you read in the introduction, as debilitating and destructive as some emotion can be, there are also clusters of emotions that carry deeply ingrained states of physiological integration or flourishing. Heartful engagement is about actively generating those. Life-generating, or heartful emotions—which are many, but include love, gratitude, hope, empathy, and compassion—carry deeply ingrained physiological- and psychological-response mechanisms just as stress and emotional chaos do. When you live a life actively engaging in heartful emotion, these new patterns are reflected throughout many of the major systems of your body and become encoded as your new "operating system."

You have learned that there is an inextricable relationship between your mind and body, and whatever "seeds of consciousness" you feed this dynamic are what you end up harvesting. Any states of emotion that you continually experience, especially ones that are deeply or routinely felt, become your life's "operating system." Heartful engagement goes a step beyond subduing your fear-response system and actively engages your calm-and-connection system; it actively pursues the development of heartful emotion.

The program offered in this book presents a specific type of mindful awareness combined with heartful engagement to lead you up the continuum of emotional integration and replace a dominant fear-response system with a calm and connected one. It is based on the steps of *recognizing, releasing, replacing, and restoring.*

RECOGNIZE, RELEASE, REPLACE, AND RESTORE

The recognize, release, replace, and restore steps allow you to effectively flip your system from one that is consumed with reactivity to one that is grounded in calm and connection. The step-by-step process is designed to bring awareness to your reactivity and emotional responses in general; subdue the reactivity's hold when it is consuming you; release the somatic or physiological buildup of your reactivity; and replace your reactivity with more life-generating response patterns. Then, through active implementation, these steps restore your emotional capacities to resilience and flourishing.

Mindful awareness, as it is applied here, allows you to recognize and then release the harmful dominance of your fear-response system. You need to recognize that you are consumed with reactivity before you can effectively take steps to reduce it. Mindful awareness invites a nonreactive state of full presence, with awareness of your emotional and physiological processes so they don't consume you. It teaches you to disengage from your typical response patterns through paying attention to your emotional attention. It is from that place of nonreactivity that you can more fully release your fear-response system's harmful buildup and replace it with different patterns of emotion.

Further, this application of mindful awareness teaches you skills to tap into a form of embodied or somatic awareness. Simply by mindfully and nonreactively tuning into your bodily processes, you are able to access deeper knowledge that might not be otherwise readily available to your more mundane conscious moments. These skills also allow you to recognize when you are dominated by a fear-response system—even down to the level of its sometimes more subtle impact.

Mindful awareness, as it is prescribed here, also teaches skills of releasing the emotional and physical buildup of your fear-response system, clearing the space for engagement in heartful emotion to emerge and be authentically possible. Heartful engagement, for it to be effective, must be authentic, and it can't be authentic if you are merely repressing your reactivity.

Once you have recognized and released the reactive and harmful impact of your fear-response system, it is authentically possible to replace the reactive states that typically consume you with heartful ones. Heartful engagement is both a state of being and a process. The process requires a step-by-step replacing of stressed-out, reactive states with heartful ones. Through engaging in this process, you will learn the power of heartful emotion in and of itself, how heartful emotion is unique to each individual, and skills in everyday life for replacing as many moments as possible with a heartful shift. Additionally, you will learn the requirement of authenticity. For heartful engagement to be transformative from an embodied sense it needs to be authentic; this authenticity creates the necessary physiological imprint for a new emotional "operating system."

Next, you will continue to replace your reactivity with a deeper level of heartful engagement through the practice of specific emotions, with an emphasis on their effective practice. Research shows the specific transformative power of gratitude, hope, empathy, and compassion, but you may be surprised to learn there are pitfalls in their practice. These pitfalls, according to research, occur when the practice of these emotions is faked, or forced—not authentically felt. The program offered here is designed to overcome these pitfalls and reap the benefits of these specifically transformative emotions.

Lastly, this process involves restoring your capacities for resilience and flourishing. Although resilience and flourishing should be natural tendencies, most of us, along the way, have never had the chance to develop them at all; or, they've been diminished through the stresses of life. The process offered here helps you achieve a deeper personal restoration through intentional heartful engagement in your everyday life. After that, the restore step takes you even further by inviting you to more fully embody your deepest values. As your life more abundantly reflects one of heartful engagement, your capacities for resilience and flourishing expand and your spiral of becoming becomes an upward one.

Through recognizing, releasing, replacing, and restoring, all aspects of the spiral of becoming are impacted; the way you perceive, the meaning you ascribe to those perceptions, and your associated physiological imprints all transform. A spiral under the influence of heartful emotions is entirely different from one under the influence of your fear-response system.

HOW A CALM-AND-CONNECTED SPIRAL CREATES CHANGE

The ultimate goal of this program is to fully engage your calm-and-connection system by the intentional cultivation of heartful emotion. In the last section, you read a brief synopsis of the steps to do just that—recognize, release, replace, and restore. Through a specific application of mindful awareness, you will learn to recognize and release the destructive nature of your fear-response system when it has run rampant. Once you have recognized and released the damaging effects of your fear response, the spaces to cultivate heartful engagement open up. This opening allows you to replace harmful reactive patterns with ones that are more conducive to emotional balance, restoration, and resilience.

Your spiral of becoming when you are in the states of balance, restoration, and resilience carries a completely different and measurable psychophysiological, or embodied, experience from when you are under the influence of your fear-response system, and you respond accordingly. Your neural, biochemical, and heart's electrical systems reflect a more integrated physiological imprint, and, if experienced routinely, those imprints cause long-term adaptations that change the nature of your emotional life. Remember, the spiral can be a downward one or an upward one depending on your dominant routine emotional experiences. Remember, also, that the spiral starts with your perceptions, progresses to the meaning you ascribe to those perceptions, and results in a physiological imprint consistent with that meaning—but then alters your future perceptions! And all this happens in a split second.

Recall what you learned about the spiral under the dominance of your fear response: it is a continual loop unless you give it a different emotional experience. That is where recognizing, releasing, replacing, and restoring come in. The steps are designed to interrupt your fear-response spiral and transform it into a calm-and-connected spiral. The goal of the next section is to demonstrate how each step of the "spiral of becoming" changes when you replace reactivity with heartful engagement.

Look back at the diagram of the spiral of becoming from chapter 1. Because the steps described above are designed to interrupt your fear response, for the purposes of explanation, we will enter the spiral as if an activating perception has occurred. In other words, we will enter in at the arrow between perception and meaning. However, because the spiral is a continuous loop, we will follow each step of the spiral all the way around to looking at how new perceptions are developed when you are heartfully engaged. This will demonstrate the transformation that occurs when you replace a fear-response-dominated spiral with a calm and connected one; or, how your downward spirals can become upward ones.

Providing New Meaning

So, imagine you have been activated by a stressful trigger. You have recognized the emotional upheaval in both your mind and body and released its hold. Now the spaces for heartful engagement have opened up, and we will look at what happens to your spiral of becoming under the influence of your calm-and-connection system. In essence, you are intentionally inviting a different emotional context—a new meaning—to your experience, transforming your fear-response-dominated spiral to a calm-and-connected one.

It is important to note here that the word "meaning" as it used in the spiral is very loosely defined. It describes the context and quality of your emotional response in that moment, or the emotional meaning you bring to it, not necessarily the meaning you attribute to the perception itself. It doesn't have to be *about*, or in direct response, to the disturbing force itself. For example, let's say I'm in a conversation with someone and I get triggered by something they say. I want to subdue my stress response and activate my calm-and-connection system so I can be grounded in the conversation, so I think about and really experience the unconditional love my dog has for me. I have intentionally changed the quality and context, or emotional meaning, that I bring to that moment without it necessarily being a direct response to the perceived trigger. The emotional meaning you bring to the moment of transition may or may not be directly related to the initial trigger.

Heartful engagement invites you to replace reactivity by providing a different and more heartful emotional experience to the moments of your life. In essence, you change the emotional meaning and context of the moment, and your physiological systems respond to the new, heart-driven experience. The program offered in this book suggests several different ways of responding to triggered perceptions that drive your fear response.

First, it could be an easy shift of awareness, as, often, your emotional attention and focus is a choice. Second, it could involve more directly targeting problematic response patterns and offering an alternative. Or, it could entail deeper rescripting of your emotional past. Finally, it could consist of addressing some of the more subtle and faulty self-images you have developed over time.

These different ways of responding are explained in detail in sections that follow. Most crucially, know that all of these ways of responding, when you are out of balance, taint your perception and contribute to the stress and emotional disequilibrium that drive your fear-response spiral. Providing a new and heart-driven emotional meaning to all these moments is the first step in transforming your spiral of becoming from stress and anxiety to calm and connection.

Creating a New Physiological Imprint

Physiologically, you are a different person when you are steeped in heartful emotion than when you are in your fear-response system. Your neural nets reflect and transform to the new experience, your biochemistry changes to reflect your integrated emotional state, and the electrical patterns of your heart respond in kind and transmit those messages back to your brain to further amplify your transformed experience. Your experience of the present moment changes as the lens through which you are experiencing life is clearer and more expansive (Fredrickson 2013b), and, because repeated experience becomes ingrained response patterns, your future also changes. Long-term adaptations occur in your psychophysiology that profoundly impact your lived experience. By actively and intentionally engaging in heartful emotions, you create adaptations in your whole mind-body complex that allow you to live life in a different way.

How Your Neural Nets Change

Recall that neurons are cells in your brain responsible for recording and transferring information. One neuron by itself does nothing; it transfers information as it connects to other neurons. Neurons connect together, forming a neural net that reflects any activity your brain or nervous system facilitates. They are what enable your brain to function and process information; they fire with everything your brain registers—a thought, a word, an experience, an emotional evaluation, the meaning you ascribe to circumstance, and so forth.

Further, the more they fire in any pattern, the better they get at maintaining those connections. However, if they no longer fire in those patterns, the neural nets actually break apart and no longer connect in the manner they previously did. This is neuroplasticity. Neuroplasticity is both the reason you may unknowingly perpetuate the faulty wiring of an overactive fear-response system and the answer to changing it.

Basically, neuroplasticity means that the connections your neurons make through your synapse patterns, and resultant wiring, are not permanent connections. They can and do change when you alter your typical response patterns. Neuroplasticity may tell you that "nerve cells that fire together, wire together," but it also shows you that "nerve cells that no longer fire together, no longer wire together." You can actually change the function and structure of your neural nets and the way they process information by breaking old experiential patterns and providing new ones. Changing your experience, including thoughts, words, meanings, and emotional evaluations, changes the connections of your neural nets and your future perceptions.

If you are your synapses, as Joseph LeDoux (2002) says, then you are a different person under your calm-and-connection system. When you bring a different emotional meaning to your life's experiences—either momentary or long term—you break the old neural connections established by previous experience and establish new ones. Neurally, you are a different person when you love than when you hate. Neurally, you are a different person when you are consumed by your fear response, experiencing stress and anxiety, than when you are steeped in gratitude or hope. More importantly, repeated connections create long-term capacities. By providing different meaning to the moments of your life by engaging in heartful emotion, you are breaking the neural connections of stress and reactivity and replacing them with calm-and-connected ones.

Also of importance is the way these neural connections are influenced by your biochemistry.

How Your Biochemistry Changes

The biochemicals of emotion profoundly affect how you feel at any given point in time, and they affect almost every cell and organ in your body. They also have their own adaptive processes that further shape who you are becoming. The parts of your brain that are evolved in emotion—the amygdala, hypothalamus, and pituitary—are also the richest areas of your brain in terms of stimulating biochemical production. They are in a constant feedback loop with either your fear-response system or your calm-and-connection system and are constantly creating the capacity for seeing and responding to life under their influence. By intentionally engaging in heartful ways of being, you reduce the influx of the maladaptive effects of unrelenting cortisol, induce the life-generating effects of your "happy chemicals," and adapt accordingly.

One of the ways this happens is through the production of oxytocin. Oxytocin is both a neurotransmitter and a hormone, meaning it is a biochemical that performs specialized functions in your brain as well as throughout your body. It is associated in both a cause-and-effect relationship with heartful emotions such as love, trust, compassion, bonding, and so forth (Zak, Kurzban, and Matzner 2005). In other words, it is produced through these emotions but also promotes more of them.

While oxytocin is not actually the opposite of cortisol, in many ways, it functions like an anti-cortisol and reduces many of its damaging effects. When oxytocin is high, cortisol is reduced. This is because oxytocin calms the amygdala (Kirsch et al. 2005). Because it calms the amygdala, it automatically reduces its influence on the hypothalamus, reducing ACTH and the resulting production of cortisol. Therefore, heartful emotions reduce your fear response and activate your calm-and-connection response; oxytocin is a primary hormone of your calm-and-connection system.

Besides oxytocin, serotonin, dopamine, and endorphins also increase under the influence of your calm-and-connection system. Serotonin is often referred to as your "feel good" neurotransmitter, and low levels have been associated with depression, anxiety, and other stress-related disorders. Dopamine its associated with your pleasure-reward centers and positive outlook for the future. It basically helps you realize when something feels good, as in positive affect, and then stimulates motivation to create more. It also contributes to creative problem solving (Ashby, Isen, and Turken 1999). Endorphins are associated with feelings of euphoria and pain relief and are often referred to as your body's natural morphine. These three chemicals, combined with oxytocin, are often referred to as your happy chemicals (Zak, Kurzban, and Matzner 2005) and are intrinsically connected to the feedback loop of your calm-and-connection system.

How Your Heart's Coherence Changes

Recall that the electrical patterning of your heart reflects your emotional state. This feedback loop sends signals of your heart's patterning up through the vagal nerve, but also stimulates more of the same. Whether it sends out signals of alert to your fear-responding amygdala and biochemical-producing hypothalamus or signals of calm is dependent on your dominant emotional state. When you are experiencing heartful emotions, your calm-and-connection system is dominant, your heart coherence patterns are smooth (McCraty et al. 1995), and this indicates a balance in your nervous system that promotes a whole mind-body response of physiological coherence. Your cortisol is reduced (McCraty et al. 1998), and you are able to further engage and develop your calm-and-connection system.

The biochemical, neural, and heart coherence states you experience under the influence of your calm-and-connection system are entirely different from those you experience under the influence of your fear-response system. When you exhibit the physiological states associated with love, gratitude, hope, compassion, and other heartful emotions, you create a physical mind-body imprint that causes momentary changes and long-term adaptations in who you are now and who you are becoming.

A New Perception

Because your spiral of becoming is a continuous loop, once you have developed a physiological imprint consistent with your calm-and-connection system or are responding to heartful emotion throughout your whole mind-body complex, your perceptions also change. You see your current circumstance through your improved embodied state, see opportunity where you before saw restriction, and experience a whole host of cognitive, behavioral, and emotional transformations.

First, state-dependent recall allows you to see through the lens of your calm-and-connection system. State-dependent recall means that when you are in a specific mood or emotional state, all the memories associated with that state have a greater tendency to surface. On the negative side, a good example is when you are in a fight or having emotional difficulty with someone. All of a sudden, you can remember everything they have done wrong in the last twenty years when, typically, those things wouldn't be in your awareness. However, the opposite is also true.

You store information in the neural networks of your brain with the associated emotional states you connect them to or what you were experiencing at the time. When associated emotional states are activated, all the related information comes to the forefront of your brain and is very present for you. When your calm-and-connection system is dominant, you perpetuate its dominance by recalling like memories, emotional states, or related information. You "see" through the lens of connection and make further choices or exhibit behaviors and reactions consistent with that life view. Again, it creates a feedback loop consistent with the dominance of that system.

Further, a tendency of seeing expansiveness allows you to see opportunity and possibility instead of the catastrophe your fear-response system deploys. When you are in any physiologically dominated state, you exhibit a thought-action repertoire consistent with that state. When you are dominated by your fear response, you have a narrowed thought-action repertoire, and when you are dominated by your calm-and-connection system, you have an expanded thought-action repertoire. What does this mean, exactly? It means that when you are grounded in your calm-and-connection system, you have thoughts and see possibilities consistent with that state, but also you expand the context in which those possibilities might exist. Further, this phenomenon plays out in your social, intellectual, behavioral, and creative life; carries short- and long-term adaptations; and increases your personal resources (Fredrickson 2013b). In short, when you are grounded in your calm-and-connection system, you perceive life in a whole different way.

When you are under the influence of your calm-and-connection system, you see expansiveness instead of restriction. This allows you to see broader behavioral options and more creative ways of responding (Kahn and Isen 1993). You are more flexible and creative, and you have a greater ability to integrate diverse material into your thought processes (Isen, Daubman, and Norwiki 1987). You see life and all your options in a broader context, your self-criticism is reduced (MacBeth and Gumley 2012), your psychological well-being is increased (Neff and Germer 2017), and you have a greater capability to undo the lingering aftereffects of an activated fear-response system (Fredrickson and Levinson 1998). You have more free-flowing choice (Fredrickson 2013a) and a greater distance from reactivity, your sense of self expands to include others in greater degrees (Fredrickson 2013a), and you have greater brain integration. When your brain is working as an integrated whole, you can better attach meaning to reason, your "thinking brain" and emotional brain are better connected, and you experience clearer decisions as well as heightened empathy and love (Begley 2007).

Lastly, targeted work with your calm-and-connection system through self-empathy and compassion can reconsolidate emotional memories and resulting perceptions, leading you to heal emotional charge around past implicit memories (Arntz 2012; Ecker 2015). You can rescript your programmed emotional triggers and perceive events from a grounded emotional state instead of one dominated by your past perceptions.

A HELICOPTER TRANSFORMED

So far in this chapter, you have been introduced to the general processes of recognizing, releasing, replacing, and restoring and how they can transform a stress-and-fear-response spiral to one of calm and connection. As an example, let us look at a specific instance of how they played out in real life—a time where I very intentionally worked to reverse the direction of an activated spiral. Although the applications and variations are considerable, this is just one example. Also, please note that although I use a somewhat more dramatic example that carries deeper ingrained reactivity, the physiological processes of a transformed spiral are similar whether you are dealing with everyday stresses or a more pronounced implicit memory. This is not meant to be a singular representation of one experience but an invitation for you to generalize to your own situations of stress and opportunities for shift.

Let's go back to the story of my son's accident and my responses to helicopters that I shared in the previous chapter. For weeks after his accident, I would experience a pronounced stress-and-anxiety reaction every time I heard a helicopter and sometimes before I was even aware I was hearing it. Maybe you have been in a similar situation, returning to the site of a difficult experience or even just an environmental reminder of a past personal conflict.

Immediately, my heart would race, and I would feel worry and begin to reexperience anxious reactions around the event. Sometimes the worry even expanded to the overall health and safety of my loved ones. Although my amygdala was doing its job well, my reactions were not appropriate for the circumstance and certainly out of context for keeping my emotional state balanced. My brain wanted to immediately take off with the chatter of what could have happened or relive the event itself, but I needed a different, authentic response to change my reactions to helicopters altogether.

First, I would recognize my reactivity. In this case, I would initially notice it by my physically felt reactions of anxiety, but it could have been more consciously driven by noticing the helicopter, recognizing my

trigger, and the immediate "chatter" that ensued. Again, the way triggers are manifested varies greatly, so the important thing is to recognize
your own patterns. I would then work on releasing the trigger's hold. As
this was a very intentional process for me, I would actually stop right
there, focus on releasing my embodied experience of stress by consciously releasing my tightened facial and shoulder muscles, and take
several grounding breaths. This releasing was foundationally important
to opening the spaces to shift my experience of helicopters altogether.

I would pause and, from my grounded state, realize that the helicopter wasn't a threat; it was the thing that actually helped my son. I then
very intentionally would cultivate and deeply feel an authentic sense of
gratitude, which I would spend several moments basking in. I then
would rest in the experiential state of the heartful emotion and let it
consume both my mind and body.

There are three very important points here. First, my response did
not have to be about the helicopter itself, and the heartful shift did not
need to be gratitude. It could have been the love I felt for my son, the
compassion of my family, or any other heartful emotion I could have
authentically felt at the moment. It didn't even need to be about the
event itself. The idea is that I was consciously trying to retrain my emotional response, not trying to debate the value of helicopters. Second, to
change my physiological imprint of the moment, and which spiral was
dominant, it had to be an authentic shift; the body knows the truth and
will respond to honest emotional experience. Lastly, it took work. It was
a very intentional emotional shift that I practiced every chance I got.

Although, obviously, I was not hooked up to lab equipment at the
time, from the scientific information presented earlier, it is a pretty fair
assumption that my physiological imprint reflected my new experience
of heartful engagement. By the shift in experience, my spiral more likely
reflected a calm-and-connected spiral than a fear-response spiral. Also,
it is important to note that I routinely and intentionally practiced this
response to incur the likely long-term adaptations from repeated experience. I can honestly say that now I still hear helicopters before anyone
else, but my immediate and authentic response has transformed; instead

of being flooded with a stress response, my immediate reaction is a heartful response of gratitude. Through intention and routine practice of heartful engagement, I was able to restore a balanced response to my original trigger and even cultivate a more generative emotional experience overall.

As you will see, the process of recognizing, releasing, replacing, and restoring has many levels and variations to address the myriad of ways you are affected by stress and emotional disequilibrium. It is designed to target the general everyday stresses you may encounter, as well as your deeper ingrained perceptions that color the lens and sensitivities of your everyday existence.

CONCLUSION: FROM FOUNDATION TO IMPLEMENTATION

Throughout this chapter, and the last, you have learned that you have two possible ways of being in the world. One is consumed and controlled by your fear-response system, as a result of the stress and emotional disequilibrium you experience; the other is thriving under your calm-and-connection system, able to be mindfully present in the world and to engage with it in a heartful way. You have learned that your perceptions translate to emotional evaluations and are expressed as physiological imprints, which become blueprints for future perceptions and behaviors. The drive that is most dominant—which, for those of us who experience stress, is the fear-response drive—is the one that controls your life.

You have also learned that when your fear-response system is in control, it must be effectively subdued before your calm-and-connection system can establish dominance. It is not as easy as just thinking your way out of the emotional chaos you are feeling because your body and brain respond and adapt to the truth of your experience, not to what you are trying to convince yourself of. If you are trying to suppress the chaos, "talk" yourself out of it, or pretend it doesn't exist, your embodied experience still remains one of stress and will adapt accordingly. Additionally, it is physiologically impossible to be in a calm-and-connected state and a fear-controlled state at the same time. The only effective way to stop the chaos of an out-of-control fear-response system and switch to a calm-and-connected system is to authentically reduce the physiological imprint of one and genuinely engage in the physiological imprint of the other.

That is where mindful awareness and heartful engagement come in. Mindful awareness is necessary to disengage, physiologically, from a fear-response system out of control. It is only from a nonreactive, nonjudgmental state of full presence, disengaged from your reactivity, that you are given the "gift of shift." It is from there you are able to shift to the awe-inspiring gifts of your calm-and-connection system. From a quieted state of mind-body connection, you can then authentically, wholeheartedly, and intentionally engage in whatever heartful opportunity may present itself. From a grounded state of open connection to love, gratitude, compassion, or whatever other heartful emotion may present itself, you are foundationally changed from the level of your cells to your lived existence.

Throughout the next several chapters, you will be applying the skills of how to effectively do this. I will walk you through the process of recognizing, releasing, replacing, and restoring. Through the skill of mindful awareness, you will learn to recognize when you are triggered, or when your fear-response system has taken control, and release its temporary hold on you as well as its long-term somatic, or embodied, buildup. Then, from a grounded and open state, you will be introduced to a step-by-step process of effectively replacing your typical ways of being with heartful engagement. You will learn the power of heartful emotions, how to identify them, and how to cultivate them. You will experience the deeper healing potential of gratitude, empathy, compassion and hope, and be invited to take all you have learned, implement it in your life, and restore your capacities for resilience and flourishing.

I know this process works; I have experienced it myself. On a day when I was frazzled and running late, stressed out with all the demands of the day, and my fear-response system was running rampant—fears of running late, fears of not being a good mom, fears of letting my students down, and more too numerous to count, I was given the gift of shift. Even when my embodied state was one of stress and emotional chaos, I was reminded of the importance of presence and full engagement. Mindful awareness brought me to a nonreactive state where I was able to be fully present. From there, I was able to recognize the awe-inspiring gift of heartful engagement. Through a heartful, engaged, and connected encounter with my dad, I was given one of the most important moments of my life.

part 2

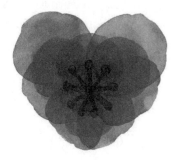

Applying the Skills

In part 1, you laid the foundation of understanding. Part 2 leads you through a step-by-step process of implementation. It walks you through the skills of applying mindful awareness and ultimately, heartful engagement so you can tangibly feel their transformative effects in your life. These skills are built on the scientific foundations explained in part 1 and are designed to develop resilience from stress and anxiety by actively cultivating your calm-and-connection system. Through a specific application of mindful awareness, you will learn to recognize and release the damaging effects of your fear-response system, and through active and intentional engagement with heartful emotion, you will learn to replace reactivity with the life-generating effects of your calm-and-connection system.

chapter 3

Recognize and Release
Through Mindful Awareness

Tara, a woman in one of my workshops, shared the following story about her transformation. It was a noteworthy story for her because it underscored the significant emotional changes she was feeling, but also their impact on one of the most important relationships in her life—the one with her mother.

One day, after Tara had been working hard to implement the skills you will learn in this chapter, she received a completely unexpected call from her sister. "I want to know what is going on!" her sister demanded. Tara, surprised and confused with the phone call and its baffling contents, answered that she had no idea what her sister was talking about. "I want to know what is going on with you—you are acting different." Still puzzled, Tara let her sister continue: "You don't fight with Mom anymore, and I want to know why!"

Tara was extremely surprised by her sister's comment and that she would both notice the shift that Tara was feeling and voice it. Her sister had noticed a distinct difference between Tara's past behavior and her current behavior, even down to the level of changing her relationship with their mother. In the past, her relationship with her mother had been quite contentious, and not much triggered her more than their interpersonal dynamics.

Tara reflected and remembered how she used to respond to the "whoosh" of her stress response in action. In the not-too-distant past, Tara had been reactive and overreactive, often lashing out when she was triggered and then hating herself for it later. Many people that knew her would describe her as an "emotional powder keg." She would often explode and say or do something she was sorry for later. She knew she needed to change, so initially, she tried to improve her behavior by just suppressing her responses. She was nonetheless triggered; she would just hold it in, either feeling like she was imploding—bottling up her reactivity and acutely feeling its chaotic effects—or having it surface later at unpredictable or misplaced times, or both. She was full of self-blame, shame, and judgment around her responses when she was stressed and needed another way. She needed skills to be authentically *nonreactive and nonjudgmental, and be fully present to her life from that state.*

As you have learned throughout this book, the sense of emotional presence you bring to each and every moment powerfully determines who you are in the moment, and also who you are becoming. This sense of presence bleeds into all other areas of your life and becomes a reciprocal system of adaptation and further perception. It is the feedback loop of your emotional life. You get better at your routine perceptions and reactions, and they then determine the nature of your transformation.

You also learned what havoc an out-of-control fear-response system can cause on your stress level and emotional equilibrium. Like Tara's experiences above, it affects everything you think, do, and say, including your relationships, and it colors the perception of your existence. When your fear-response system is running rampant, you cannot effectively cultivate a sense of calm and connection—an embodied state of emotional integration, resilience, and flourishing. You must first appease an unsettling fear response before you can actively cultivate the opposite.

So far, you have reflected on the global and far-reaching role stress and emotional disequilibrium may play in your life, identified some of your personal triggers and the nature of your personal inner chatter, and looked at how stress and emotional upheaval may manifest in the physical sensations of your body.

In this chapter, you will implement a specific type of mindful awareness to recognize and release reactivity, in your mind and body, subduing the dominant nature of your stress response. First, you will reflect on your trigger points, learn to identify when they are consuming you, and learn the "Power of Pause"—a mindful and intentional way of disengaging from your reactivity so it doesn't consume you. Next, you will expand your mindful skills by learning to pay more acute attention to where your attention is focused and the impact of training your awareness to be grounded in the present moment.

Further, sometimes your stresses or emotional triggers are somewhat veiled in your everyday life and either surface at unexpected and inappropriate times or remain below the surface and cause emotional or physical unease. It takes more intentional mindful awareness to allow them to surface and be released. Accordingly, you will engage in activities designed to do just that—in both mind and body. You will dialog with and release emotional buildup from your thoughts; dialog with and release somatic, or emotional, buildup from your body; and work on releasing buildup from your body exclusively, as, often, destructive emotions get lodged there and need physical release as well.

UNDERSTAND YOUR TYPICAL RESPONSES

However, before we begin, it is important to name and bring an awareness to what your typical reactive patterns might be if you are not mindful of them. This recognition both helps you not fall into your automatic response patterns as well as better distinguish and differentiate what a mindful response is. So, what are the typical ways you might respond when your stress response is triggered? First, you might take off with the reactivity, in an emotional sense, and allow it to consume your awareness in both body and mind. This, you have learned, only exacerbates your stress response and furthers the downward direction of the spiral of becoming.

Second, you may try to suppress it, pretending it doesn't exist, or assuming if you suppress it enough, it will go away. You may confuse suppression with nonreactivity. Nonreactive means that you are authentically disengaged from the emotional impact of your typical reactive response, not merely suppressing it. Suppressing doesn't work; when you try to suppress something, it is still being experienced throughout your subconscious mind and your embodied response. It may surface later masked as something else. Your body and your subconscious mind know and will reflect your emotional truth, whether you want to admit you are experiencing that truth or not. Simply put, suppressing is not mindful, and it is not effective. Third, you may blame, shame, or judge yourself for having the reaction because if you were evolved enough, you wouldn't be having the reaction that is consuming you, right? You feel guilty because you are experiencing "afflictive" emotions, and afflictive emotions are "bad." Self-blame, shame, and judgment carry their own inherent problems and just further your stress spiral in a downward manner. As you will see shortly, mindful awareness is a fourth, much more effective option.

Tara tried all these approaches at one time or another, and none of them worked for her. It wasn't until she learned to apply the skills of mindful awareness that she was able to effectively subdue her triggers and be present for her mother in a whole different way.

Your progression of mindful skills to recognize reactivity starts with transforming your response to overt reactivity—the states of reactivity that are all-consuming and demanding your attention. Those are the states most pronounced and easy to detect—the volatile states in your everyday awareness that cause you to react or overreact, often before thinking. The reactions may be external, causing stress-colored reactions, behaviors, or choices, or they may be internal, where you absorb their harmful emotional impact in both your mind and body. You are consumed with the internal experience of stress without necessarily reacting. Both exacerbate your stress spiral, and you need another alternative.

RECOGNIZE OVERT REACTIVITY

Mindful awareness invites you to have an awareness of your reactivity without your typical stimulus-response patterns emerging, which is a very different way of responding than merely pretending the patterns do not exist. Recognizing, pausing, and discerning are the necessary components to pacifying an overtly reactive system.

So, what do you do when your reactivity is an obvious and overt fear response vying for your attention? What happens when your reactivity is so strong it highjacks you throughout your body and mind and you have an all-consuming response? Sometimes the mechanisms of your fear-response system are so pronounced they literally take over your whole mind-body complex. What do you do then?

Bring to mind chapter 1 when you learned about the dynamics of your fear-response system. Recall how it is the amygdala's job to send out an all-consuming alert when it senses danger, and its interpretation of what danger is is based solely on programming from your past experience. Remember also that it provides conscious and subconscious meaning to all you encounter and has you perceive through the lens of any past threat, imagined or real, and it does its job very effectively. It is trying to keep you safe from what it deems has been harmful or threatening to you in the past, even if it is as off-base as an errant helicopter. It is a fire alarm in your brain being activated when there is not necessarily a fire.

Fully recognizing your reactivity without immediately responding to it requires awareness, and your awareness in this area can be trained. Refer back to the Identifying Emotional Triggers activity in chapter 1 and feel free to add to it or edit it as you see fit. Coming into a fuller understanding of the stress and emotional upheaval in your life is a fluid process, and as you progress, you may realize that it impacts greater areas of your life or plays out in ways you weren't originally aware of. The idea here is to take some time thinking of situations, events, people, and so on that are the likely areas to stimulate a reactive response in you.

Coupled with what you learned about the amygdala, you can begin to recognize these patterns when they are activated and anticipate when they might show up for you. You may even want to broaden your understanding of these triggers and the far-reaching effects in your life. When you are aware that these triggers are under the auspices of your amygdala, it is easier to be aware of their presence without necessarily taking off with their reactivity, and mindful awareness invites you to do that. Remember, your amygdala is the "watchdog" of your safety, but it may be barking needlessly. In the above example, Tara learned to recognize when her amygdala was active, observe her reactivity from an emotionally disengaged place, and even experience some humor at its diligence.

Recall also that when you are triggered, you experience an all-consuming physical response. In chapter 1, you identified typical ways you might experience the physical reactive patterns of an activated fear-response system. You can train yourself to recognize that these physical reactions are an indication that your fear response has been activated and with the knowledge of how the whole process works, not succumb to its take-over. When you can understand and embrace the beauty of your fear-response system without having to surrender to its high-intensity alarm every time it is activated, you have already begun to lessen its impact and develop a nonreactive posture toward it. You can even learn to appreciate your reactions for how they have tried to protect you in the past, at the same time realizing that they may no longer be serving you well.

After reflecting on what you originally identified as your triggers and physical-response patterns, and armed with the additional information you have learned since, can you see how they may play a broader role in your life than you previously identified? Can you see that with awareness of the process, you can begin to identify when they are active in your life and cultivate a different stance toward them?

Mindful awareness invites a nonreactive, nonjudgmental awareness of your emotional triggers, a distancing from their emotional impact. It is as if you are observing your reactivity from an emotionally disengaged point of view without being consumed by it. Once you can identify and recognize your reactive patterns when they surface, engaging in the Power of Pause helps you cultivate a nonreactive posture in response. In the earlier example, learning to pause was the pivotal turning point for Tara. Instead of responding and overreacting in her typical ways, an authentic, nonreactive pause allowed her to chose an intentional response.

LEARN TO PAUSE

The Power of Pause is a holistic mind and body response to reduce the impact of reactivity by cultivating a nonreactive stance toward it. Armed with the information on how your fear-response system works, as well as knowledge of your own broad areas of triggers and physical responses, you can learn to pause before reacting in your typical ways. The pause itself begins to break the neural chain that usually carries you from one reaction to the next, quite often resulting in full-blown psycho-physiological chaos. Not only does it break the chain of reactivity, it begins to rewire a different way of responding to life's triggers overall and establishes more grounded response patterns. Additionally, the Power of Pause reduces the reactivity of every stage of the spiral of becoming. The meaning you assign to a perception is from a clearer, more grounded lens; your fear-driven biochemical impact is reduced; the electrical patterns of your heart are not as reactive; and the neural nets of further reactivity are subdued, allowing you to further perceive your situation differently.

The Power of Pause is learning to recognize your reactivity without being swallowed up by it. You can stay mindful and aware of what is happening inside of you without allowing it to consume you. As you learned earlier, sometimes you hear mindful awareness being referred to as "becoming the observer" or "cultivating the witness," as if it were someone else's experience you are observing. Those terms are used to describe a way of "being with" something from a nonreactive disengaged point of view. The Power of Pause invites that way of responding right in the moment of reactivity. The Power of Pause is an indispensable step in reducing the impact of your fear-response system and laying the foundation for replacing your stress response with emotional resilience and flourishing. The practice itself will be presented shortly; however, before you learn the practice, it is helpful to identify situations where you are likely to benefit from its use.

Exercise and Reflection: Implementing the Power of Pause

Being aware ahead of time of situations where you might benefit by using the Power of Pause, as well as the specific benefits you may incur, helps remind you to use it in the reactivity of the moment. They may be similar to the triggers you just reviewed, or in addition to those, but here, you are focusing more on the specific situations in which those triggers may manifest. The more situations you can be mindful of now, the more likely you will remember to use it when the time comes. Remember, also, that changing a reaction in the moment can profoundly change the outcome of a situation overall, possibly leading to life-changing moments.

1. List many situations in your own life, big and small, where you might benefit from taking a moment to pause.

2. What systems can you set up now to remind yourself to use the Power of Pause when the time comes?

3. What benefits overall might you incur from its use?

4. What benefits to specific situations might you realize?

Process and reflect in a stream-of-consciousness type of writing.

Once you have identified situations in which you might benefit from using the Power of Pause, it is important to actually implement it. Often people cognitively know what they "should" do, but don't actually implement the strategies for change. Remember, it is experience that transforms. Your first contemplative practice is called the Power of Pause—the actual implementation of an intentional shift in reactivity.

Practice: The Power of Pause

The Power of Pause invites you to pause in the moment of reactivity and adopt a different posture toward it altogether. It invites you to simply pause, recognize the trigger from a nonreactive stance almost as if you are observing it from a third-person point of view, and refrain from evaluating it or its emotional significance. It is an "in-the-moment" practice, meaning you can do it any place and time you want to cultivate a nonreactive response to your triggers.

When you are triggered in your mind or body or both, do the following:

1. Recognize the trigger without engaging in it, evaluating it, or suppressing it.

2. Disengage from its emotional and somatic (or bodily) hold, as if it were someone else's experience. Become the observer and be with it from a nonreactive, nonjudgmental stance.

3. Take several very intentional breaths, including intentional sighs if it feels comfortable to do so, and let your awareness settle on the experience of breathing.

4. When you can begin to feel your reactivity subside, reassess the situation from the grounded state of the pause.

What were your experiences practicing the Power of Pause? Was it effective for you? Could you remember to practice it when you were triggered? Did your responses and interpretations of the moment change?

Practice three to four times a day for the next week and record your experiences. There is a downloadable practice record log available online at http://www.newharbinger.com/42839. I encourage you to download this log and record every time you engage in one of the practices and your experience with it. As I stated in the introduction, recording your responses to the practices offered in this program is an important component along your path from stress and anxiety to resilience and well-being.

From reflecting on your triggers and engaging in the Power of Pause, you have learned to recognize overt, or obvious, reactivity and respond in a different way. However, sometimes it is hidden in the natural rhythms of the day; it is there from an observable sense but may need your awareness to acknowledge its presence. This requires paying attention to where your emotional attention is in the first place, in both mind and body. As you refine and deepen your skills of mindful awareness, you will now turn to your more subtle patterns of reactivity.

RECOGNIZE THE POWER OF YOUR ATTENTION

Recall how neural programming works. Anytime you place your attention anywhere, be it on a thing, a thought, a feeling, or an impulse or word, the neural networks in your brain fire in response, record the experience, and establish patterns. Remember, your neural networks are mechanisms of information flow and records of experience (Siegel 2010). Wherever your attention is directed determines your associated firing patterns. To make matters worse, you may not even be aware of the focus of your emotional attention. You may have become so accustomed to the repetitive and negative nature of your estimated sixty to eighty thousand thoughts a day that you are largely unaware of their existence. Recognizing reactivity sometimes requires focused attention.

Also, remember the Feeling States of Awareness activity you completed in chapter 2. Certainly, your physical and psychological states were impacted during the initial events you wrote about but, in all likelihood, they were impacted by just bringing your attention to the event as you were writing about it. You likely experienced the same physiological and psychological responses by merely *thinking* about the event. Your attention creates a mind-body response consistent with its emotional nature, even if you are not fully aware.

You are constantly embodying every momentary experience, physiologically and psychologically, through your directed attention, and transforming accordingly. And, as much as your attention matters, you might not even be aware of its focus. If you are like most adults, your focused attention is likely anywhere but the present moment. You might be thinking about all the things that are going wrong, playing conversations in your head, or experiencing the loops of inner chatter you wrote about in chapter 1 and not even realize it!

Bringing awareness to your attention is the first step in being able to recognize the subtler influences of your fear-response system. Many times, it may be in your control, and you might not even be aware of it. By bringing your attention to your attention, you can begin to recognize your habits of more subtle reactivity that may before have gone unnoticed. Attention to attention is different from recognizing your obvious triggers or emotional highjacks, as those are much more obvious and dominate your conscious experience. Paying attention to attention invites you to recognize your more indirect or elusive habits of thought that may have a much greater impact on your emotional equilibrium than you realize. Further, once you gain the skills for this type of awareness, you can better identify when future patterns of stress are beginning to emerge and disengage from them before they take control.

The insights of bringing your attention to your attention can be surprising and informative. You may have not known something was bothering you so much or occupying so much of your emotional attention. You may gain important insights about issues you need to deal with when it is appropriate to do so. If you can take note of where your attention is without letting it consume you and notice if any issues need further attention, promise yourself you will go back, and deal with them when the time is right, you often then are able to disengage from their emotional hold.

Paying attention to attention involves both your cognitive, or conscious, attention as well as your bodily sensations. The insights you can gain from bodily awareness are equally important and the process similar. You might not even notice you are tightening your shoulders, are clenching your teeth, or have uneasiness in your stomach. Just like the insights gained from mental attention, these can carry important information about your underlying emotional landscape.

As you further your skills of mindful awareness, you are now invited to look at the more subtle impact of your everyday attention and the objects of your focus. Mindful awareness invites full presence, and an important step to cultivating that presence is noticing where your mental and physical attention is in the first place. The following activity is designed to bring your awareness to the focus of your daily attention and the power it holds over your emotional experience.

Exercise and Reflection: Paying Attention to Attention

This exercise asks you to pause several times a day and reflect on where your attention is: what thoughts you are thinking, the things you may be ruminating on, the stories you are telling yourself about your circumstances, the things you are anticipating, and so forth. It also asks you to reflect on whether the typical focus of your attention allows you to be truly present with what is going on in the moment and identify reactivities you may be experiencing beyond your conscious awareness.

1. Make a plan to pause several times in the next day or two and notice where your attention is. You might set up a system to remind yourself by setting a timer; putting a sticky note on your rearview mirror, a mirror at home, or somewhere else you often look; or pausing every time you touch a doorknob. The idea is to just stop for a moment and bring your awareness to your attention, the words you are saying to yourself, your consuming thoughts, and your feelings and physical sensations.

2. After you have taken notice for a few days, write in a stream-of-consciousness style addressing some of the following questions. Remember, the questions are not meant to be answered verbatim; they are only to guide your thinking.

  1. Where is your attention typically focused throughout the day?

  2. What are your thoughts and feelings focused on?

  3. What stories are you telling yourself about your current circumstances?

  4. Are you typically fully present with what is going on, and, if not, how can you become so?

  5. Besides bringing your conscious awareness to only your thoughts, what is your body telling you by its demeanor?

Pause and reflect in a way that is appropriate for you. What did you learn about the focus of your attention? Did you discover any insights or surprises?

Once you have spent some time just noticing the nature of where your attention is, next you will work on skills to bring yourself fully present—the next step in mindfully recognizing and reducing your stress response.

BECOME PRESENT

Mindful awareness invites you to be fully present. Recognizing where your attention is, both mentally and physically, helps you become aware of the nature of your presence and shift it accordingly. If, when you bring your awareness to your mental and physical attention and you find

you are distracted with worries about the future, negative interpretations of the present or anxieties about the past, you are offered the "gift
of shift." In those moments of recognition, you are offered the opportunity to recognize where your attention is without blame, shame, or judgment; receive any important insights; and intentionally bring your full
attention and awareness back to the present moment.

When you are able to bring your full attention and awareness to the
present moment, you begin to break the typical stimulus-response patterns that you are accustomed to. Your neural nets begin to break the
connections of your typical reactions and rewire to less reactive ones.
Further, because you are not reacting in your typical ways, your ingrained
fear response begins to subside, and there is a physiological settling in
your whole system. Lastly, maintaining this presence further allows you
to recognize or be aware when new triggers or emotional challenges
surface, and to retain a nonreactive stance toward them.

Your next practice is called Present-Moment Awareness. Although
deceptively simple, it is profound in its ability to break typical attentional chains of thought and reaction and bring you truly present to the
possibilities of the moment. Pausing and becoming present were the first
and necessary things I needed to do that morning with my father. If I
had not first become present, I would never have been able to engage
with him the way I did.

Practice: Present-Moment Awareness

The practice of present-moment awareness is also an in-the-moment
practice, meaning you can do it any place and time you want to get
grounded or remain grounded. It only takes a few minutes, although
you can remain in this state of mind-body awareness for extended
periods of time with practice. It invites you to first recognize where
your attention is, both mentally and physically; note if there are
present issues you need to address at a later time; commit to do that;
and disengage your attentional hold. Once you disengage your atten-

tion from where it was, you bring it fully present to the moment you are experiencing. You are not consumed with worries about the future, anxieties about the present, or regrets about the past. It often helps if you can hyperfocus on your physical senses, your immediate surroundings, or both.

1. Notice where your attention is, physically, mentally, and emotionally, and disengage from its hold.

2. Relax the muscles around your eyes, shoulders, and chest, and take a releasing breath or intentional sigh.

3. Continue to breathe comfortably and naturally as you bring your attention to your immediate environment and your physical senses.

4. Pause and *experience* your senses, including the sights around you, as if you are hyperaware of the encounter. Notice what it feels like to be fully present.

5. Maintain this state of awareness as long as is comfortable or appropriate.

Practice Present-Moment Awareness three to four times a day for the next week. Record your experiences in your practice record log.

What was this experience like for you? Did this sense of presence feel different from the typical sense of presence you bring to your everyday moments? What did you learn from engaging in the practice, and what adjustments might you make?

Cultivating present-moment awareness allows a quietening of the mind and body. It allows you to cultivate a sense of full presence where you are not consumed with stress, anxiety, or triggers and helps to subdue your fear response. Practicing this type of awareness cultivates your capacity for a deeper presence more often and helps you better recognize and watch for stress in your life going forward, as you consciously arrest stress states before they become fully manifest.

Sometimes, however, if you are not fully able to recognize and disengage from harmful emotions or an out-of-balance fear-response system as it happens, you can harbor the residual effects, and they need to be released. Learning to release reactivity throughout your mind and body is the next step to dissipating the effects of a dominant fear-response system.

RELEASE REACTIVITY THROUGH YOUR MIND AND BODY

Your mind and body may harbor residual effects from pent-up and harmful emotion, which sustains and worsens your fear-response dominance. These residual effects, then, need to be released, or they can cause long-term damage. This "hanging on" happens in both your mind and body, although, as you learned earlier, one or the other may be the dominant modality. It is important to understand this because that is the modality that needs to be targeted for release. More simply, sometimes this releasing can be done through a primarily cognitive process, and sometimes it requires directed somatic releasing.

Release Through Your Mind

Following is an exercise and reflection activity, Writing for Release. It is based on a writing process to mindfully release some emotional residue you may be harboring, through an emotional-cognitive process. The idea is that emotions that are not recognized or processed initially become trapped in both your mind and your body, and writing about them releases them and externalizes them so you can let them go.

This exercise encourages you to write about fairly recent events that you feel you may still carry some emotional charge around. The process, as it is proposed here, is meant to be approached with a mindful and "observing" attitude, disengaged from reactivity, as if it were someone else's experience. You might even observe with a little curiosity or amusement at their intensity. In other words, it is not meant for you to relive and reexperience events; it is meant for you to recognize that they are still there for you and release their hold. (Also, although it may look similar to something called expressive writing, which encourages writing about significant traumatic events [Pennebaker 2018; Balkie and Wilhelm 2005], writing for release is not that, either. Issues of deeper healing will be addressed later in this book.)

Like the other writing exercises proposed in this book, Writing for Release is also meant to be done in a stream-of-consciousness style not concerned with grammar, sentence structure, or spelling. Let the writing freely flow; you may find that, as you write, you have access to much more emotional content than you realized. My dear friend Dr. Habib Sadeghi has developed a similar process he calls Purge Emotional Writing or PEW 12 (Sadeghi 2017). The "12" means he suggests that you do it for twelve minutes. What I love most about the way he suggests doing this writing is that you burn it when you are done, underscoring the idea that this type of writing is meant to bring up the residual emotion, release it, and let it go.

Exercise and Reflection: Writing for Release

The writing is meant to be done for only ten to twenty minutes and is meant for emotional release. It is okay to stop writing at any time if you feel you are reliving rather than releasing. Exercise some self-care and take note as it might be something you want to focus on as the book progresses. Also, it is not meant to be a cerebral or rational process. You might not even have an idea of what you will be writing about before you start. It is as if you are letting the writing lead you, and you are observing the process with an open awareness.

1. Find some paper other than a notebook dedicated to the reflective writing here and a timer you can set for ten minutes.

2. Find a quiet place where you can get centered and will be uninterrupted for ten to twenty minutes.

3. Do the Present-Moment Awareness practice presented earlier in this chapter for two to three minutes.

4. Set the timer for ten minutes and simply begin to write whatever comes up for you, originally without prethought about content. The idea is you are providing an open awareness for emotions to emerge, not consciously directing your writing. Rest in and be present to whatever emotional cues surface for you, and start writing with an openness and acceptance, even if it seems like jibberish. Try and keep your pen to the paper, or your fingers to the keyboard, to prevent the voice of the "inner critic" from popping in your awareness. If you have trouble beginning, just start randomly writing and see where it leads you, as if you are observing the process. Some people, if they feel stuck beginning, write with their nondominant hand. It is theorized that nondominant handwriting helps to bypass your analytical thought process and more freely access emotion. Remember, your job is to be fully present to yourself with a disengaged, nonjudgmental open awareness.

5. At the end of ten minutes, discern if you are done or if you would benefit from another ten minutes.

When you are done, you are invited to burn the paper in a safe place and as immediately as possible. However, if some important insights came up for you, it is okay to keep it. If you are called to burn it, when doing so, rest in the felt sense of release.

What were your experiences with this exercise? Did some surprising emotions or past experiences surface for you? How do you feel now? Are there some lingering questions or thoughts you have about what you wrote about? Process and reflect on what you learned by engaging in the activity.

In the activity you just completed, you brought mindful attention to allowing pent-up thoughts and emotions to surface and be released through a mindful thought process. Sometimes, however, your body is a more effective mode of access because it has more direct access to your subconscious mind. The idea of working somatically, or through your body, to access emotional information is that attention, or mindful awareness, to physical sensations can help the subconscious become conscious. In other words, by focusing on your physical sensations, you enable your brain to access emotional information that was previously beyond your immediate awareness.

Release Through Your Body-Mind

The impact of your somatic experience is subtle. Earlier in this chapter, you were introduced to the word somatic, or the concept that you reflect your psychological or emotional experience throughout the systems of your body. "Somatic" means primarily experienced through the body, although the body and mind can never be truly separated in the reflection of emotional experience. When emotional experience is expressed somatically, it is often sensed as a bodily knowing, often immediately beyond the description of words, although words may come later if gently persuaded.

While you may have more obvious somatic responses when noticeably triggered, like the physical reaction patterns you identified in chapter 1, you also have very subtle somatic responses. Your everyday attention, conscious mind, and subconscious plays itself out in all the systems of your body. Because your body is more connected to your subconscious mind than your conscious mind is, going to your body for answers is an effective tool in sensing emotion beyond your awareness. Like everyday conscious attention, everyday somatic expression may go largely unrealized without your focused awareness, yet its impact can be powerful.

Again, you adapt to every momentary experience creating greater capacities for more of the same, and subtle but harmful somatic experience is no different. Because of the mind-body feedback loop of adaptation, even subconscious somatic experience can contribute to an out-of-control fear-response system. More simply, if you carry it in your body, you carry it in your mind, even if you are unaware, and if it is dominated by your fear-response system, it is contributing to a downward spiral of your emotional life.

Bringing awareness and attention to your physically felt, or bodily, circumstance is somatic mindfulness. It is a powerful type of attentiveness you can bring to your somatic, or bodily, sensations that can reveal emotional connections and help verbalize their presence. Being mindful of the subtle sensations throughout your body gives you a different lens of perception to your emotional experience. The power of attention is not only conscious; it is also somatic.

By bringing your awareness to your bodily sensations, sensing what they feel like and being open to the experience, the neural networks of associative memory enable your conscious brain to take in the sensory information and begin to mediate a response. In other words, your brain accesses the previous "association" of the neural networks of sensation with the neural networks of an emotional memory and begins to process it in a conscious way. It associates the somatic experience with the emotional memory and brings it to conscious awareness. It is your body's own way of finding its way to cognitive expression through your intentional open awareness of bodily sensations. Further, if you "listen" closely enough, your bodily sensations will tell you if your cognitive evaluation is an honest expression of your experience.

What does all this mean in easily understandable terms? Your body reflects all your emotional experience through its intimate connection with your subconscious mind. By resting in those sensations, you can enable the subconscious emotional information to become conscious. This information can often reveal for you if your fear-response system is activated, and, frequently, it can reveal why. In essence, you are letting your body lead in an awareness of your emotional attention, a powerful tool in recognizing your reactivity.

The following exercise is designed to help you recognize the nature of your emotional experience through somatic awareness. It is built on the foundation of a therapeutic practice developed by Eugene Gendlin (1981) called Focusing, although the practice presented here is different. In this exercise, you are invited to dialogue, through writing, with your somatic sensations and see if they carry a useful emotional interpretation or an ability to better recognize your emotional landscape.

Exercise and Reflection: Somatic Dialoging

Somatic dialoging allows you to communicate, in a sense, with your bodily knowing. If you pay enough attention, you may be able to recognize that somewhere between your conscious and subconscious, there is a region of knowing that is expressed and recognized through the sensations of your body. Eugene Gendlin referred to this as a felt sense. This felt sense is often manifest as unclear inner sensations that can initially appear vague, but with gentle awareness and prompting, it can develop into a fully conscious yet novel or intuitive way of understanding. Somatic dialoging doesn't come from a cognitive space of trying to figure something out; it comes from a gentle space of letting a different kind of information emerge. Further, in staying true to the roots of the practice of Focusing, the language is intentionally general. It is important that you let the somatic sensations of your body guide your process without too much cognitive analysis.

1. Find a space and time where you can sit quietly, get fully grounded, and bring a gentle awareness to your body.

2. Take several deep breaths and discharge any overt emotional reactivity.

3. Settle into a deep and quiet awareness of your body and notice if any physical sensations become evident. Remember, somatic dialoging is about letting your body tell you, not the other way around. Your job is to be a patient, quiet, fully engaged listener.

4. When a physical sensation appears, ask if it has a
    message for you, and be fully open to receiving its
    message without analysis. Notice if any images, intuitive
    knowings, or other nonspecific information emerge.
    Don't push too hard or overthink it; remember, you are
    merely trying to gently coax what may feel murky into a
    more defined awareness.

5. If an image, a more defined sensation, or other
    nonspecific information emerges, gently sit with it and
    see if the original sensation shifts a bit. This is how your
    body responds. You will feel an "intuitive yes" if you are
    on the path to revealing the emotional truth that may
    lie beneath the sensations. It is a delicate dance between
    the emerging sensations and images, your receiving, and
    further testing your embodied response for validity—
    but when the original felt sense shifts in its bodily
    expression, you know you are on the path to discovery.

6. Keep with this process until you feel a noticeable shift in
    bodily sensations and a better cognitive understanding
    of their message. In other words, often, when you come
    to a conscious and emotional understanding of what
    is beneath the surface of your somatic awareness, you
    will feel a shift in bodily sensations; they may shift in
    placement, lessen in intensity, or diminish altogether. It
    is often experienced as that moment of aha!

After you have spent some time in somatic dialoging with the
sensations you feel, write in a stream-of-consciousness style to
process your experience. You can use the writing as an extension of
your dialog or even as the tool to help you receive the information in
the first place, as if you are in conversation with the felt sense. The
writing, connected with the dialoging itself, can be a powerful combination in consciously recognizing what your body already knows.

The next step of releasing the impact of your fear-response system throughout your whole mind-body complex is to focus on the trapped residual emotional impact on your body exclusively.

Release Through Your Body

There is a substantial amount of burgeoning research that shows you can somatically trap the results of emotion that is not fully recognized or processed (Van der Kolk 2014; Ogden, Minton, and Pain 2006). While much of this research is done on trauma, the underlying concept is true for lesser emotional difficulties as well. The theory behind this research is that if not fully processed, the results of unresolved emotion get stuck in your nervous system and need a release mechanism (Levine 2010). The feedback loop of your fear-response system is constantly assessing your somatic state, or bodily sensations, and sending messages back to your brain about your degree of emotional well-being.

Because so much of your emotional life is an embodied experience, paying attention to and releasing residual somatic buildup is essential for emotional equilibrium. You have sensory nerve fibers throughout your body called interoceptors. Interoceptors receive and transmit sensations originating from the interior of your body. They sense what is going on for you internally and transmit that information to other parts of your body to adjust accordingly. When your body is in a state of equilibrium, they work hard to maintain that equilibrium. However, if your body is out of somatic balance routinely, or for too long, they either can't respond effectively or they sense that your body must need its stress resources elevated and further transmit those messages.

This hyperarousal increases your access to emotionally difficult or traumatic memory through state-dependent recall (Van der Kolk, Van der Hart, and Miramar 1996), and your system remains dominated by a profound and consuming fear response. Releasing at the somatic level changes the information your interceptors receive and pacifies your whole mind-body complex. In essence, you are jumping in at the physiological imprint level of your spiral of becoming. By releasing your fear-activated response, your interoceptors, instead of continuing to send an alert response, send a different message to your brain, and it responds with an appeased assessment of fear or threat.

Following is a practice for somatic release. It is based on the concept that through the combination of interoceptors and afferent nerve fibers—the nerve fibers that deliver messages to your brain—you can intentionally subdue your emotional system by calming your body. More simply, interoceptive nerve fibers detect bodily sensations, and afferent neural pathways are the pathways that lead information to the brain. Essentially, these nerve systems work together to sense what is going on in your body and tell your brain how to perceive that activity and respond accordingly.

We usually think of certain muscle activities, for instance a smile or tension around the eyes, as a reflection of emotion, but they are also producers of emotion. The muscles associated with emotion are in a continual feedback loop. They physically respond to how you are feeling, but you can also use them intentionally to tell your brain how to respond with the corresponding desired feeling. Again, you are jumping in at the physiological imprint level of the spiral to reverse its direction from a downward one to an upward one. The muscles associated most with emotion are your facial muscles, specifically the ones around your eyes and mouth and the larger muscles throughout your neck, shoulders, spine, and hips. So, too, is your diaphragm, the muscle in your abdomen that controls your breathing. Also, while you can intentionally relax specific muscles, you can also nudge them into a greater relaxed state by progressively tightening and then releasing them. Progressive muscle relaxation has been shown to subdue a heightened stress response by lowering cortisol, heart rate, and blood pressure (Kim, Na, and Hong 2016).

Practice: Somatic Clearing

The practice below provides for somatic releasing through releasing specific muscle groups known to be associated with emotion. You can follow the instructions on the list by memory, record yourself reading the narrative, or access the associated audio file, available online at http://www.newharbinger.com/42839. You may want to play relaxing music in the background.

Find a comfortable place where you can lie down for approximately twenty minutes uninterrupted, and do the following:

1. Let your awareness find your breath at a focal or still point somewhere in your torso that is comfortable for you. Take several releasing breaths, repeating the word "release" on the out breath and physically feeling the sensation of release throughout your body. Maintain this type of breathing for several minutes, continually releasing deeper and feeling your body becoming heavier, as if it were melting into the surface below you. Keep this pattern of breathing throughout the practice.

2. Bring your awareness to your eyes and spend some time releasing all the tiny muscles surrounding them. Do the same with the rest of your facial muscles. It might feel as if you are letting go of any expression on your face.

3. Release all the tightness throughout your shoulders, and bring your focused awareness back to your chest and your released breathing.

4. Starting at your toes, progressively tighten for a three-count and then release the following muscle groups: your lower legs from your toes to your knees; your upper legs from your knees to your hips; your whole torso, front and back; both arms simultaneously from your shoulders to your hands.

5. Now, imagine a wave of release starting at your toes and very slowly and systematically coming all the way up through your body, creating a profound release as it passes each area.

6. Bring all your awareness back to your breath, as if your body has melted completely into the surface below you. If it feels comfortable to do so, cultivate a tiny smile.

7. Rest in this state for the remainder of the twenty minutes.

After practicing the somatic clearing exercise described above, record your experience in your practice record log. How did it feel? Were you able to feel a physical and emotional shift? How do you feel right now in an emotional sense? How might you incorporate this practice in your life to reap its benefits? Process and reflect in a way that is appropriate for you. This is also a rich time to journal, as often through a somatic release, new emotional insights open up.

CONCLUSION: CLEARING THE WAY FOR HEARTFUL ENGAGEMENT

Recognizing and releasing through mindful awareness pacifies both your mind and body. It subdues your fear-response system and stops the spiral of becoming from spinning out of control. It allows you to use your conscious awareness to be mindful of your entire mind and body experience without placing value on it or judging it. This nonreactive fully-accepting presence stops your typical stimulus-response patterns and allows a new openness to emerge. It allows you to recognize your triggers and physical reactions without succumbing to them, judging them, or suppressing them. It allows you the Power of Pause. It shows you how cultivating a present-moment awareness can ground you in the present instead of leaving you to ruminate on the past, suffer anxiety about the present, or worry about the future. It helps you recognize when new stresses may be surfacing, and it helps you release emotional toxins from both your mind and body, opening up possibilities for another paradigm to emerge. It teaches you how to dialog with the innate wisdom of your body and learn truths that may otherwise have remained buried, and it helps you release residual somatic toxins and balance your system physically. Most importantly, through an embodied approach to recognizing and releasing through mindful awareness, you open up the spaces for heartful engagement to emerge. With a subdued fear-response system, your calm-and-connection system has room to enter and flourish.

In the next chapter, you will be learning and applying the skills of heartful engagement. You will learn what heartful engagement feels like for you from an embodied sense and be able to distinguish the heartful emotions that are strongest for you. You will learn easy skills of implementation and practices so you can foster it in all the moments of your life, as well as sustained practices to cultivate it at a deeper level. As a result of recognizing and releasing through mindful awareness, you now have a system ready for the calm and connection of heartful engagement.

chapter 4

Replace Reactivity with Heartful Engagement

Teri was terrified to go in and talk to her boss. She knew "terrified" seemed like a strong word to describe how she felt, and she probably would not have used that word aloud verbally, but inside, that is exactly how she felt. She was shaking intensely, her heart was racing, her chest was tight, and her mind was screaming. She felt like she was all alone in her struggles and that certainly everyone else she worked with must have a better handle on dealing with him. You see, he was one of "those people." He was so stressed-out himself that he continually made it everyone else's fault, and everyone in the office dreaded to come into contact with him. He created an environment of toxicity wherever he went. Although she knew he was a problem with everyone, and on an intellectual level knew that she was just one of many, emotionally, she felt like she was being singled out and, for sure, everyone else in the office must have it more together and handle it better. Yes, terrified is what she felt— even knowing that the feeling on the inside was far out of proportion for the circumstance. And, consistent with how most people struggle with stress, she felt alone in her experience.

Worse, the more she thought about it, the more agitated she felt, the worse it got, and the more alone she felt. All morning, she was playing out in her head all the dire scenarios that were sure to happen. The more she catastrophized, the worse she felt, physically *and emotionally, and the worse the scenarios got. She was panicked in mind and body, and she felt like she had a ton of rocks crushing her chest with their weight. She began to recognize her response patterns were far out of context for the situation and was even able to pause, become present and quiet, and release some of their hold on her. She was able to recognize and disengage from the triggers she was experiencing in both her body and mind and began to feel her system being appeased. Although she felt somewhat better, without an alternative focus, the destructive thoughts just kept coming back. She needed something more. She needed to replace the crazy thoughts in her head with ones that would nurture a whole different response so she could see opportunity instead of restriction.*

You have learned so far in this book that there is an inextricable relationship between mind and body, and whatever you feed this mind-body dynamic as the "seeds of consciousness" are what you end up harvesting. These seeds of consciousness become your primary operating system and determine the way you perceive and function in the world. You have learned that to effectively reduce the stress and anxiety in your life, you must subdue your fear-response system and actively cultivate your calm-and-connection system. You have experienced how a specific form of mindful awareness can help you recognize and release your reactivity and open the spaces for a different paradigm altogether— a paradigm that opens the spaces for heartful engagement to emerge.

Engaging in heartful emotions—for example, deep love, connection, compassion, gratitude, and so forth—can literally unite and transform your brain, your heart, and all the cells in your body. By experiencing what these heartful states are like inside you, you can activate the dormant impulses of them, cultivate them, and embody them, resulting in an integrated sense of well-being. If you do so intentionally and routinely, you activate your calm-and-connection system, it becomes the primary operating system of your mind and body, and your baseline interpretation of life adjusts to higher levels of happiness. You feel more integrated and grounded, and you see more opportunity and feel more expansiveness (Fredrickson 2000 et al.; Fredrickson et al. 2008; Zeng et al. 2015).

This chapter is about understanding and applying the beginning skills of heartful engagement to replace the stressed and anxious states you have learned to recognize and release. It introduces concepts, skills, and practices that will intentionally activate your calm-and-connection system throughout your body and mind. Through a process of written activities and active implementation, you will ever deeper develop your capacities for heartful engagement and integrated emotion. You will begin to feel a shift to the expansive free-flowing state that is characteristic of peace and well-being and is the opposite of stress.

The trajectory offered here starts with understanding the requirements of intentionality and authenticity in heartful emotion and its individual nature of experience. From there, you will identify your own experience of emotion and learn simple skills to begin to replace stressed-out states with heartful engagement. Building on those skills, you will deepen your experience through HEART, a practice designed to help you intentionally engage heartful emotion so you can regulate your *affect*—your embodied or experienced emotional state.

ENGAGE HEARTFUL EMOTION

To rewire your stress response through an embodied approach, it takes an active, intentional, and authentic engagement in heartful emotion. The neurons comprising your fear response are faster and more numerous than those of your calm-and-connection system. They had to be for our species' immediate survival. But with the stresses of our current culture, they have been overactivated to an unhealthy level. And you need to intentionally engage the neurons of your calm-and-connection system—by pursuing moments of love, connection, compassion, or whatever is a genuine heartful emotion for you—in order to rebalance this scale.

It's also true that for heartful emotion to truly be transformative, it must be authentic. Remember, you are not consciously trying to talk yourself into a different emotional experience; you are transforming your emotional system at the level of your neural nets, biochemistry, and heart coherence. Your body knows the truth of your experience, not just what you think you should feel or want to will into existence. For heartful emotion to transform you, it must be a genuine embodied experience reflected throughout the physiological systems of your body.

This section offers you a step-by-step process to pursue just that. First, it is helpful to gain some clarity on the individual nature of emotion semantics, or understand the diversity in how people experience emotion, and the resultant embodied experience. From this understanding, you can more easily identify what, for you, are embodied heartful emotions or the ones that you experience the deepest. After you have a grasp on your individual experience of heartful emotions, you can develop the beginning skills for their implementation and begin to see their benefits.

UNDERSTAND DIVERSITY IN EMOTIONAL EXPERIENCE

Specific emotions aren't experienced the same way for everyone. In other words, what may be a heartful emotion for you might not necessarily produce the same response in another. Using an embodied approach, we define emotion as helpful or harmful by the physiological state it incurs—whether it activates a fear response or calm-and-connection response. This is consistent with both Dan Siegel's definition of emotion as "degree of system integration" (Siegel 2009) and Neil McNaughton's theory that emotion ought to be classified by the biochemical state it produces in each individual, rather than by universal classification (McNaughton 1989). Using this approach, we can see that some emotional experiences can be life-generating and transformational by the physiological state they produce, and some can be life-depleting—but they are different for everyone.

We see this in the fact that the same emotional words can produce different results in different people. Why might one person beam at the thought of love and another cringe? How you learn and store meaning around emotion is dependent on the emotional and embodied state you experienced when you learned the meaning of the word. Or, if you had a powerful contradictory emotional experience, even after you learned the concept, the experience could override your original learning. What does all this mean in practical terms? If you were told you were loved and you were abused or neglected at the same time, the term "love" would take on a different embodied experience for you. You might think in your mind what love *should* mean, but your felt experience of the word would likely be decidedly different. To make matters worse, you then may beat yourself up because you don't feel the same in response to the word "love" as many people around you do. Of course, that all exacerbates your complicated embodied experience with the word.

Let us imagine Teri from the example in the beginning of the chapter. She needed an alternative heartful emotion strong enough to not only reduce her fear response, but to replace it with feelings that would ground her in her own essence. When I asked Teri which emotions felt most heartful for her, she originally put love at the top of her list, but she found she couldn't really practice it. She had just gotten out of a relationship with someone who cheated on her even as he professed to love her. So, she had an embodied experience of the word that was in conflict with what she thought the emotion *should* mean. Forcing herself to feel it because she thought she should brought up the imprint of self-judgment because she wasn't truly feeling love at all. What might have been a more truthful embodied emotion for her at that moment would be to rest in the compassion she had been shown at a pivotal time in her life. In other words, emotions, for you, are the truthful experience of them.

Another good example is the word "forgiveness." Many, many people have found profound healing from employing forgiveness and would feel, and physiologically express, the corresponding imprint. Others may not be ready to forgive because they have not healed enough personally around what needs to be forgiven or feel they still need some recognition of the hurt before they can move forward. The reasons aren't important, and this isn't meant to be a discourse on forgiveness; however, it is important to understand that the embodied experience of those people would be vastly different. Further, the self-blame, shame, and judgment around not feeling like you think you ought to carry an even more pronounced life-degenerating physiological imprint.

I once had three women in a workshop debate whether the term "potential" symbolized a heartful emotion or not. For one woman, it was a strongly heartful word because when she heard it, she could deeply connect with all the beautiful things she aspired to be. For her, it symbolized shining hope for her future, and she could powerfully feel the associated embodied experience. It was an important word. Another woman hated the word because much of her pain came from feeling like she had never lived up to her parental expectations, and the phrase "You're not living up to your potential!" felt like a dagger to her heart. The third woman had very little emotional attachment to the word in any way, and although she could understand on a cognitive level the other women's experiences, hers carried no embodied response at all. Three women, three different embodied experiences of the same word.

This is an important concept to absorb as we move forward. It is not the accepted definition of an emotion that is important as much as it is your individual response patterns. A heartful emotion, for you, is any emotion that elicits the biochemical, neural, and heart-pattern changes consistent with your calm-and-connection system. As you learned through the spiral of becoming, they produce life-generating physiological imprints that create your capacities for more of the same. These are the ones that, for you individually, create greater states of embodied integration, complete with the biochemical, neural, and heart patterns to match.

How do you know whether an emotion is heartful for you? You know it when you feel it. Just as "stress" is an umbrella term that pertains to anything experienced as emotional disequilibrium, heartful emotions are experienced by a felt sense of emotional integration. The experience of these emotions facilitates embodied states that are often characterized by phrases such as "being in your Deepest Self," being in the "flow" or in the "zone," and "grounded in your center." However you characterize them and whatever phrases you use to describe them, you know them when you feel them. At this point, it is not as important to debate definitions or which emotions are heartful or not as it is to recognize and define for yourself which emotions create an embodied state of "felt integration" in you. Rest in your body; let it tell you. And honor your experience without blame, shame, or judgment.

Exercise and Reflection: Emotional Charting

You are going to use the following chart to discern what, for you, are generative and heartful emotions, or related concepts, and what emotions are degenerative. In your journal, draw a horizontal line halfway down a fresh page. Write "generative emotional experiences"—ones that give you a felt sense of integration, resonance, or coherence—above the line, and "degenerative emotional experiences" below the line. Assign a height value for your embodied experience of each: the more heartful they are, the higher they should go on the page, and the more destructive, the lower.

Remember, what you're listing here are not things or situations, but the feelings that certain things or situations bring up for you. The feelings you list are not meant to be listed in columns or ordered in any way, except assigned a height value for intensity; you should brainstorm freely, writing the feelings down all over the page. For instance, above the line, for me, I might write love, compassion, connection, serenity, gratitude, hope—any emotion that gives me a sense of authentic groundedness and clarity, not fleeting or shallow emotional responses. Meanwhile, below the line, I might write disconnection, worry, anxiety, fear, insecurity, guilt, and so on—emotions that are reactive and keep me from really, freely living. These, too, would carry a felt sense—but one of uneasiness, agitation, anxiety, or disconnection. Finally, I would assign a height to each emotion based on how they affect me and what kind of deep felt sense they provoke in me, with the most generative at the top and the most degenerative at the bottom.

Again, let your embodied experience of the exercise guide you, not your cognitive appraisal. Write as quickly as you feel comfortable to access your intuitive sense when writing. Notice if you are critical of what you are writing and pause to remember to be authentic to your own experience. Above all, remember: *there are no right or wrong answers.*

Let's process what the chart reveals for you. For now, let's just look at what you wrote above the line. Process and reflect why these states hold importance for you, what situations bring them present for you, what they mean to you, and how you feel when you experience them. Were there any surprises? Did you notice if you felt you *should* write something you didn't really feel? Did you judge yourself for anything you felt called to write? Explore, now in a narrative sense, what emotions are most heartful for you, where you experience them most in your life, and what they feel like when they are most embodied. Write in a stream-of-consciousness style and engage this exercise on a deep level, as these felt-states will be used as a foundation of understanding throughout the rest of this text.

There is a lot to be learned from this chart, and throughout the next chapters, you will revisit it often. Remember, the trajectory here is designed to have you start with basic understanding and implementation and work at ever deepening your experience.

Look at the top of the chart and the words you listed above the line. Just by definition of the way I asked you to write them down, they are life-generating. In other words, all the physiological responses that you gain from cultivating these states create adaptations that lead to deeper capacities to live in those states more often. Simply put, they begin to rewire your stress response from one of fear and anxiety to one of calm and connection. These are the ones that, for you individually, carry the biochemical, neural, or electrical changes associated with generative transformation. Choosing to intentionally cultivate these states begins to transform you all the way from the level of your cells to your lived experience.

But what does this list of heartful emotions specifically mean in terms of your day-to-day life? And how do you begin to live your life to more often reflect them? The three-to-one ratio and micromoments, which are explained in the next sections, are the beginning and foundational steps to experience the effects of heartful emotion. They help you identify and experience states of heartful emotion in your day-to-day life; they are your introduction to the concepts of intentionally shifting your emotional awareness and what that new experience *feels like.*

Although, as you know, I tend to shy away from labels of "positive" and "negative" because of the judgment inherently placed on the negative, there is huge overlap between the concept of positive emotions and the concept of heartful emotions. We can extrapolate a lot of understanding from the research done on positive emotion because both definitions share many emotions, and to do so, we will revisit Barbara Fredrickson's work on positive emotions.

EMPLOY THE 3:1 RATIO OF EMOTIONAL TRANSFORMATION

Fredrickson's research on the influence of positive emotion shows that a three-to-one ratio of positive moments to negative moments can make a profound difference in your transformational process (Fredrickson 2013b). It shows that looking at all your moments from this point of view, the day-to-day and moment-to-moment choices you make, literally causes you to see, behave, react, and live in your world according to how those moments accumulate. Although she also says that a four-to-one or five-to-one ratio gains even greater benefits, the three-to-one ratio is the critical tipping point. I find this ratio a helpful and tangible tool because it makes the whole idea of transforming your daily choices doable. In other words, it is not human nature, nor emotionally honest, to try to be in heartful states 100 percent of the time. This ratio gives you the idea that if you can just tip the scales of your emotional attention and be intentional about creating more life-generating moments than not, big shifts can take place. Also, it is based on research on real people, in real life, making significant transformations.

Let us look at how these concepts may play out in your everyday life. First, remember that every moment of every day, you carry a physiological imprint that reflects your emotional state of that moment and transforms to the imprints most often and most deeply experienced. The idea behind the three-to-one ratio is that you are reflecting a life-generating imprint often enough for it to be the dominant mold or pattern. Second, remember that you reflect and mold to the authentic emotional state you are experiencing, not what you think you should feel, what you are trying to force yourself to feel, or what might be a genuine heartful emotion for someone else but, for whatever reason, isn't one for you.

I find it helpful to use the emotional charting exercise you just completed in conjunction with Fredrickson's three-to-one ratio. Keeping the above concepts in mind, look over your chart and reread the reflection you wrote about it. What moments of shift are possible? How do you meet that ratio? You will be asked to write and reflect on some of those ways shortly, but first, it is important to bring your awareness to the power and impact of *attentional choice* and your ability to create *extra moments* through intention that will help tip the scales.

Many times, your emotional awareness is a choice. For example, I may be driving to work or walking across campus, and my emotional awareness can just as easily be focused on all the things in my life I am grateful for or on merely appreciating my surroundings, as it can be focused on all the negative inner chatter that usually accompanies most of our moments. Instead of obsessing on what has just happened or worrying about what is going to happen, I could be fully present and connecting with my surroundings and the people in them. Think about the exercise you did in chapter 3, Paying Attention to Attention, that asked you to notice where your attention was at various points of the day. Now, think about the Emotional Charting exercise for a moment and consider that many of the moments when you are focused on something below the line may be a choice of focus, a habit of thought. Think about all the opportunities of "shift" that the day offers. When you can use the chart as a reference for what heartful emotions are for you and visualize shifting above the line as much as authentically possible, you may realize that you have more control over your day-to-day awareness and transformation than you previously thought.

Another important tool is the realization that the three-to-one ratio doesn't need to comprise moments already occurring in your life. In other words, you can create those moments intentionally. In Fredrickson's research, she has identified something she calls micromoments. These are small moments during the day that you can purposefully create to tip the scales of the ratio.

CREATE MICROMOMENTS OF CONNECTION

Micromoments are exactly as they sound: small moments of intentional and heartfelt connection throughout the day. You can create them by momentary choices of behavior, for example giving a genuine smile or gesture of appreciation, laughing, appreciating the beauty around you, or recognizing someone for something they are doing well. Such moments are not necessarily ones that would happen without you being purposeful about them, yet they are also not major events that you need to create. Sometimes, they're happening around you already, and all you need is to consciously and mindfully absorb them as they happen rather than staying on automatic pilot and letting them pass you by. Remember the Present-Moment Awareness practice in the last chapter. Micromoments invite you to bring mindful awareness to those moments and then intentionally engage with whatever heartfelt connection that moment offers. However you experience micromoments of connection, they are powerful tools in the smaller moments of your day to create the bigger shifts that transform your existence from one of stress and anxiety to one of resilience and well-being.

I was conducting a workshop once, and a woman raised her hand and shared that she was convinced by everything I was sharing but was at a loss on how to really "do it." "Am I supposed to wake up tomorrow and just be totally different?" she honestly asked. No. But remember, as a "system of adaptation," you are constantly transforming to every moment of every day. And in the world of neuroscience, little changes add up to big differences. What you do on a micro level, over time, becomes who you are on a macro level.

How do micromoments transform you? Although there are many, one of the important ways this happens is through oxytocin. As you learned in chapter 2, oxytocin is a hormone associated with your calm-and-connection system. Oxytocin is both a result of your behavior and contributes to more of it. It can be produced in little spurts all day long that can lead to profound changes. Imagine yourself with an oxytocin IV bag on your arm all day. Every time you pause for a genuine encounter, share a smile, have a meaningful conversation, pet a dog, or appreciate the beauty around you, it is like you are giving that IV bag a gentle squeeze and providing opportunity for your calm-and-connection system to flourish.

Beyond oxytocin, as you have learned, every time you have an experience, the neural nets in your brain reflect that experience. The more you have any experience, the more your neural nets form to a greater capacity for that experience or like experiences. Micromoments of connections are little shifts interspersed throughout the day that have a big impact on your neural activity in both function and structure. This means that momentary function of your neural activity shifts, but so does the structure of these nets, creating long-term change. Simply put, the way you perceive your present situation changes, as does the way you perceive your future.

Exercise and Reflection: Apply the Ratio and Create Micromoments

Refer to the Emotional Charting Exercise and Reflection. Building on the general concepts you identified in those exercises, what are specific and concrete ways you can tip the three-to-one ratio in favor of heartful emotion in your daily life? How can you create micromoments of connection throughout the smaller moments of your days? Use stream-of-consciousness writing to process and reflect in a way that is appropriate for you. Identify as many situations as you can think of and how you can intentionally and authentically engage in the opportunities.

NOTICE THE BENEFITS

The benefits you will gain through heartful engagement will continually deepen. They will become more pronounced in your life, both as heartful engagement becomes routine practice and as you progressively deepen your application of it. However, it is also important to recognize some of these benefits as they are beginning to appear in your life, as your conscious awareness of them can also help foster their growth.

Research has shown substantial and numerous benefits of the practice of heartful and positive emotion. Heartful and positive emotions can undo the undesirable effects of negative emotion and regulate their impact (Fredrickson and Levinson 1998). It has shown that they can increase resilience, positive social experience, and your sense of well-being (Emmons and Crumpler 2000). They have been shown to buffer against depression and increase positive subjective interpretation of experience (Harbaugh and Vasey 2014). Their practice has also been shown to increase your sense of expansiveness, connectedness, resourcefulness, and your thought-action repertoire, which basically means broadening your ability to see solutions to problems (Fredrickson 2013b). And these are just a few of the many benefits.

Exercise and Reflection: Note Your Shifts

As you begin to implement the skills of heartful engagement in your everyday life, take notice of any shifts that may occur, and briefly record them in your journal. Notice both small, everyday occurrences—for instance, you might find shifts in the way you perceive certain things; maybe something that has bothered you in the past may not be so dominant anymore—as well as bigger shifts; maybe your overall demeanor has improved or you are becoming more resilient to difficulties. Keep in mind the above list of benefits documented by research, but don't limit your experience to what was listed above; just notice when an upturn of awareness has occurred for you.

Ultimately, this is best done as an ongoing reflection as you continually employ the practice of heartful engagement. How you record your moments of shift is up to you. You might want to make a note of them as they happen and keep an ongoing list, or you may want to reflect daily or weekly on anything that you have noticed. It is just important that you do take note of them as they begin to occur.

Now that you have the foundations of what heartful emotions feel like and how to make an intentional shift in your day-to-day life, you will focus on deeper application. Beyond heartful engagement in everyday awareness, research has shown substantial benefits from directed practice. Because you adapt to experience, the deeper, more intentional, more often, or longer you engage in heartful emotion, the more it transforms you. But how do you effectively do that? A major component of this program is HEART.

As I shared earlier, HEART stands for *heartful emotion affect regulation training*. HEART is a threefold process of noticing experience; refocusing your physiological response (releasing the tension that is a hallmark of the embodied imprints of stress, relaxing your breathing, and grounding your awareness); and finally, nurturing heartful emotion to bring on the corresponding embodied imprint of calm and connection. It is designed to regulate your affect, or replace destabilizing emotional states with the emotionally integrated states of resilience and well-being.

HEART can be adapted to many contexts; you can use it in specific moments of reactivity to cultivate more general and heartful states of mind or as a standalone meditative practice to come into deep contact with a heartful, calm-and-connected state. It is an important foundation of the rest of this program, and the variations of HEART get progressively deeper and more directed as they advance. Following is an introduction to these practices and the first of the series.

HOW HEART WORKS

Again, the basic steps of HEART are *notice*, *refocus*, and *nurture*. They are very generally based on the first three concepts of the overall program presented in this book—recognize, release, and replace—but are much more specific in their design and implementation. An explanation of each step and a brief description of its physiological impact follows.

Notice

Pause, turn inward, and ground yourself in your torso. Take a few grounding breaths, and from a disengaged, witnessing, observing, or third-person point of view, notice what your thoughts are without letting them consume you. Notice how diligent or frenetic the activity of your mind might be. Without suppressing them, feel your thoughts fade in intensity as you bring yourself back to your breath. Then notice what you are feeling—which may or may not be associated with your thoughts. Notice if what you are feeling comes from a different place in your body than your thoughts, and notice its texture and strength without being consumed. Again, just notice without judgment. Then notice any bodily sensations. Notice if those sensations carry with them an underlying feeling or message.

Physiological implications. In this step, you break the chain of your typical reaction patterns. You slow your body's stress response, quiet your neural nets, reduce your cortisol influx, and begin to improve your heart's coherence.

Refocus

Release all the tension in the tiny muscles all around your eyes. Release all the tension in the muscles surrounding your shoulders. Let your awareness drop to a place in your torso that feels comfortable for you, and focus on slow, natural, comfortable breaths at that focal point. Extend your out-breath a bit longer than your in-breath and continue to absorb your awareness in breathing.

Physiological implications. Your eyes have a direct neural connection to your amygdala, both by what your eyes see, but also by detecting the muscle tension in the muscles around them. Again, your bodily sensations and muscles associated with stress are in a constant feedback loop with your deep brain. Your muscles respond to your brain's triggers, but then further your stress response by their state of tension. You can jump in at the physiological level of the spiral of becoming by releasing the tension around your eyes, this feedback is sent straight to your amygdala, and your whole emotional system begins to calm.

Releasing the tension in your shoulders further calms your stress response, and your attention on a spot in your torso reduces your racing thoughts. Bringing all your awareness to your breath further reduces your cortisol and activates your parasympathetic nervous system, which is the nervous system that calms your whole body. From this calm state, you are now more receptive to an authentic and embodied shift to heartful emotion.

Nurture

(This step is the most varied in HEART and depends on the intention of the practice. A generic description follows.) Intentionally shift to an emotional state that, for you, carries a felt sense consistent with the heartful emotions you identified earlier. For many people, an image helps bring up the felt sense. If this is true for you, hold this image in your awareness, notice what it is that makes you feel the emotion, and, as deeply on you can, experience the emotion from an embodied sense. Continue the breath pattern you established earlier, and continue to rest in the experiential state of the emotion for as long as is comfortable, as long as you can sustain it, or whatever time limit you have set for yourself. If you find yourself jumping from image to image, don't worry; it is not the image that is important; it is the embodied state it cultivates. Focus on the felt sense with whatever image or images work.

Physiological implications. This step is where you actively cultivate your calm-and-connection system. Your neural nets now fire with the new experience. Oxytocin, along with other generative biochemicals are produced—serotonin and dopamine—your parasympathetic nervous system continues its dominant shift, and your heart coherence levels rise consistent with your embodied experience. Your biochemical shifts and heart rate variability patterns are sent back to your brain, which continues the feedback loop, and your calm-and-connection system becomes dominant.

We have learned an important lesson in actively training our calm and connection system from the discipline of positive psychology. Positive psychology is the branch of psychology that has a primary focus of studying human flourishing rather than mental illness. It teaches us that transformation more readily occurs when you don't just reduce what is wrong but intentionally create what is right. HEART is about intentionally creating the emotional states you do want, rather than just reducing those you don't want. With HEART, you train your system by actively and intentionally engaging in heartful emotion, as a directed practice, often enough, deep enough, and in crucial moments so that deeper physiological transformations can take place. And I say "practice" deliberately, because HEART is like exercise; you need to do it often to train yourself for the intended result. Done right, HEART promotes the deeper rewiring from stress and anxiety to resilience and well-being.

Now that you know the basics of HEART, let us see how it might play out in your everyday life. How, for instance, might you use HEART right in the moment of reactivity?

HEART IN THE MOMENT

When you do HEART right in the moment of reactivity, you rewire your responses as they happen. The major benefits are twofold. First, it has the potential to completely change your response in that moment. The benefits of this cannot be overstated. How many times have you reacted in a situation in a way that was not good for you and yet had to suffer the possibly long-term and serious consequences? Second, the more often you stop your triggered reactions as they are happening, the

more you rewire a newer, less reactive response altogether. You are actually reducing your neural capacities for reactivity.

HEART in the Moment, which is described in the next exercise, is
a simple technique to use—but you'll need to do a little reflection first
to identify when you'll engage the process and which heartful emotions
and embodied experiences you'll focus on when you do.

1. Refer back to the Emotional Charting exercise you did earlier
    in this chapter. Pick a few of the heartful emotions you identi-
    fied that you feel you might be able to access fairly readily.

2. For each of those emotions, try to think of some images that
    would bring up the felt experience of that emotion. Write them
    in your journal. Write down a variety of images, as different
    levels of reactivity will respond to different images.

3. Finally, list as many situations as you can think of for which you
    think you'd benefit from using HEART in the Moment.
    Identifying reactive situations ahead of time increases the likeli-
    hood that you'll remember to use the practice when you need to.

Once you've done this work to prepare, you'll be ready to practice
the technique.

Practice: HEART in the Moment

1. *Notice* your reactivity in your thoughts, emotions, and
    bodily responses and disengage from it or witness it.

2. *Refocus* your physiological response by releasing the
    muscles in your eyes and shoulders, dropping your
    attention to your torso, and establishing a grounded
    breathing pattern.

3. *Nurture* the felt and embodied experience of a heartful
    emotion, possibly holding an image in your mind and
    heart as you do so. Soak in the experience.

Let us go back to Teri as she practices HEART to see how this plays out in real life.

Teri was terrified to go in and talk to her boss. Because, in the past, the interaction with him had been difficult, she knew she needed to be clear-headed, so she practiced HEART in the Moment. She noticed her racing thoughts but began to disengage and observe them as if they were someone else's. She noticed her feelings and recognized fear and insecurity. She also noticed they were located in her chest and upper torso. Naming them helped her distance their hold on her. She also witnessed but disengaged from a pit of dread in her stomach. She took a breath, released her eyes and shoulders, and focused on a slow breathing pattern at the level of her solar plexus because that is what felt comfortable for her. She remembered her emotional chart and the word "compassion." When she thought of that word, an image emerged of a teacher she had in elementary school who comforted her one day when she was very upset. Teri imagined herself bathed in the compassion of this woman and imagined her teacher's arms surrounding her and a bubble of protection surrounding them both. Teri immediately felt a shift and was now much more grounded for the meeting. She even imagined her teacher and the bubble of compassion in her boss's office with her. This all happened in less than a minute, but Teri was a different person going in to that meeting. Once in there, her calm and empowered state deflected his combative one, and the meeting was noneventful.

Teri talks about her shift in the meeting as nothing short of amazing. When she went in, her boss was his typical self: berating and condescending. Teri was different, however. Resting in the heartful emotion of compassion she had cultivated before she went in and really feeling its effects, Teri was able to just let her boss's hurtful comments and negative attitude fall away; she described it as feeling like Teflon where nothing he said "stuck." Her heartful emotional state empowered her, and because her attitude was different with him, he softened in his delivery because he wasn't met with the typical resistance or upset from her and pushed off balance in his own response.

Practice HEART in the Moment at least four times in the next week and make sure you are recording and reflecting on your experiences in your journal. You may want to reflect on some of the following questions, answering the ones to which you feel called. How did it feel? Were you able to remember to do it in moments of reactivity? Were the outcomes of the situations changed or softened? Were the emotions you used effective in that situation? Is there anything you would change in the future as you engage in the practice? Make sure you record your continual practice as, the more information you have, the more successful the practice will become.

Practice Variation: HEARTful Outlook

HEARTful Outlook follows the same basic steps as HEART in the Moment: you notice reactivity mindfully, refocus your physiological response to open space to engage your calm-and-connection system, and deliberately nurture the experience of a heartful emotion. However, in the nurture step, you engage an emotion that is the opposite of the stressed one you're feeling. This is designed to replace a specific problematic attitude with one more conducive to resilience or well-being in that particular moment.

For example, let's say you were about to give a speech, and you were very nervous. Practicing HEARTful Outlook would invite you, during the nurture step, to feel and breathe a sense of confidence, to directly counteract the nervousness that might be challenging your emotional balance. The difference in HEARTful Outlook is that it is designed to counteract a specific and challenging mindset with another, more emotionally grounding one.

Michelle was a workshop participant and had struggles in her relationship and lacked confidence in her work. She was particularly drawn to the in-the-moment practices because she would often react or feel an overactive fear response in the moment, and perceive all her situations from that lens. Following are her words about HEART in the Moment and the variation of HEARTful Outlook:

HEART in the moment was very successful for me. I used the image of my dog's face mostly. Her unconditional love for me triggers feelings of love and happiness. At first, I thought it would be easy, but to do it right, you cannot trick yourself into feeling a certain way. The first time it happened, it was such a trip. It was so weird, I could actually feel it alter my body and my perceptions. I would describe it as a feeling of elation, and you can actually feel when you do it right. I used it a lot in different situations, and the time that stands out most was during a fight I had with my husband. I told him I had to go to my "happy place" for a moment. It really worked! I actually came up smiling. I tried HEARTful Outlook before a presentation one day when I was feeling super nervous. I just "breathed" a sense of calm, and it helped me get centered. I think these practices work so well for me because they are so in the moment.

In-the-moment practices are indispensable for changing your reactivity, your reactivity patterns overall, and the possible outcome of the moment. However, sustained practices create the length of time and depth of experience necessary for more substantial change.

SUSTAINED HEART: STRENGTHEN YOUR HEART MUSCLES

Sustained HEART is a contemplative variation on the notice, refocus, and nurture process in which you create and maintain an inner focus centered on a deep experience of heartful emotion. While in-the-moment practices rewire your moments of reactivity, "sustained" practices—which are exactly as they sound, practices that you hold for sustained periods of time to lengthen and deepen your experience—create foundational changes in your baseline emotional make up (Fredrickson et al. 2008).

Here, we'll devote some time to considering the images you'll use in Sustained HEART—which may differ from the ones you use for HEART in the Moment. In your journal, complete the following tasks.

1. Revisit the emotional charting exercise. Look at the emotions you wrote above the line and see which ones stand out for you in a way that you could hold them in a deep sense of heartful engagement for a sustained period of time.

2. List some images that would bring up those emotions for you, remembering again that the images may shift and change, but the important thing is the felt experience. These are similar to the images you would use during the nurture step outlined earlier but could use for a more sustained period of time.

Now, while ample benefits have been documented from various sustained contemplative practices, the biggest impediment is getting people to actually do them; planning ahead for success increases your likelihood of adherence. Remember, experience is the thing that transforms you, and the only way your practice can do that is if you actually engage in it often enough for change to take place. The conditions under which you practice greatly influence your habitual engagement, and setting these conditions before you begin helps lay the foundation for success. As you think about the following conditions for success, it might be helpful to keep in mind that a sustained practice means you will be engaged in the practice for a period of time and is best in an environment where you can fully focus. After you learn the conditions that contribute to a successful practice, you will be walked through the practice itself.

All in all, designated space and time for practice are the biggest predictors of success. Some people have a dedicated space in which to practice, complete with a personal altar and a specified time every day to practice. However, if you have less personal space or a busy life, you may need to be creative. My first practice space, many, many years ago, was in a transformed closet. I often tell my workshop participants or students that even five minutes in a parked car will do a world of good. Be creative, find what works for you, but the more thought you can put into it ahead of time, the more likely you are to stick with it.

Consider the questions below and write a few paragraphs on how you will implement a sustained practice. Be specific. This is an important piece as the program advances, as many sustained practices will follow.

1. Given the current state of your life, what space can you find for your practice?

2. How will you build it into your schedule? (Five to fifteen minutes a day will produce some positive changes. Twenty minutes a day will produce even greater benefits.)

3. Would you prefer a silent practice or one with ambient music?

4. Would you prefer a guided audio?

5. What kind of support do you need?

Practice: Sustained HEART

Sustained HEART lays the foundation for all the HEART practices throughout the rest of the book. It follows the generic steps of *notice*, *refocus*, and *nurture* as outlined above but is designed to be done at a deeper level for a sustained period of time, so each step is expanded for depth and breadth. The explanation of the practice is more at length here, as the specialized variations you will engage as the book progresses builds from it. You can commit the steps to memory, record them, or have someone read them to you. Sustained HEART is, as are all the longer HEART practices throughout the rest of the book, available as a guided audio if you prefer to have me walk you through the practice. You can find the audio online at http://www.newharbinger.com/42839.

Begin by sitting comfortably in a position you can maintain for a sustained period of time.

Notice your thoughts, emotions, and body sensations and disengage from their hold. The notice step in Sustained HEART is similar to HEART in the Moment; however, you might not be having any obvious reactivity. The notice step in this practice asks you to take a brief inventory of the mental, emotional, and physical states of your body.

Take a few intentional breaths and begin to establish a natural and calm breathing pattern. From the point of view of the witness, or observer, notice any thoughts or mental activity you might be having. Again, don't let the thoughts take you away or engage in them; you are just witnessing or observing them.

Next, notice your emotional activity. Your emotional activity may or may or not be associated with your thoughts. Are there any feelings that stand out? Are your emotions harbored in a different spot in your body than your thoughts? Again, you are just noticing or observing your emotional activity and its nuances without letting it consume you. You're not "thinking about" as much as you are just "being with."

Now, notice the physical sensations in your body. Are your shoulders or any other areas of your body tight? Do you feel anxious? Scan your body. How does it feel? Are any areas harboring stress or tightness? If you feel stress, tension, or tightness anywhere in your body, make a conscious effort to release it. If it feels right, you can also begin to repeat the word "release" silently on the out-breath and imagine yourself releasing all the tension from your body.

Refocus the physical tension in and around your eyes, your shoulders, and your torso. Breathe. The purpose of the refocus step is to refocus the physical attributes of your body to bring you deeper into the experience and make you more receptive to the next step. The two main parts are first, refocusing and releasing through the eyes, the shoulders, and the torso and second, deepening your breathing.

As you continue to ground yourself in your breath, focus your attention on your eyes, and release all the tiny muscles around the eyes and the eye sockets. It might feel as if you're losing the expression on your face. Again, you can continue to repeat the word "release" on the out-breath if it feels comfortable to do so. If you are repeating the word "release," physically feel the sensation of release throughout your body every time you repeat the word. Now release any tension, tightness, or stress in your shoulders. With every out-breath, physically feel the sensation of release a little bit more acutely. Now, bring all your awareness to an area in your torso that feels comfortable for you. It could be your heart; your solar plexus, which is right below your heart; or it could be deep in your belly.

Now, deepen your breathing. When you are at the breathing step of Sustained HEART, your conscious attention is keenly focused on an area of your torso that feels comfortable for you and on the process of breathing. Again, this is where some people really find it helpful to focus on the word "release" on every out-breath and vividly feel the sensation of releasing throughout the body. Some contemplative traditions recommend you count each breath. In Sustained HEART, during the refocus step, you might find that helpful.

If you choose to, count each in-and-out cycle as one breath. Many people count from one to ten and then go back to one, while others count from ten down to one and then go back to ten. The idea is not to count how many breaths in total you are taking, for example ending at 565; it is to engage your mind just enough not to have it on a hundred other things. Counting your breaths is just a tool to keep your awareness focused on your interior process and further let your body settle. Again, if your attention is keenly focused on your breathing, it won't be on anything else.

The main concept to remember in the refocus step is that you are physiologically readying yourself to deeply engage a heartful contemplative experience.

Nurture a deep experience of a heartful emotion. Once you begin to feel a deepening of your physical experience, make a conscious and intentional shift to a heartful emotion. The main goal of this practice is that you maintain a heartful emotional shift long enough and deep enough that you begin to make foundational shifts in your whole mind-body complex. It can't be faked. It can't be forced. Sincerely felt heartful emotion creates physiological, biochemical, and neural response patterns that are very real and very powerful and create profound change if you practice regularly.

While keeping an intentional breath somewhere in the background of your awareness, shift your attention to something that engages your heart. This could be an image that you listed in the last exercise, something that sincerely generates "felt states" above the line on the heartful awareness chart, or something that is currently more heartfully present for you. It could be reexperiencing a time when you have felt it before, or what you imagine it would feel like.

If using an image helps you to create or maintain this engaged state, it is a good tool to use. However, it is important to remember that the image is just a tool, and a genuine heartful focus is the most important aspect of this practice. Occasionally, I have participants who, theoretically, have something above the line that they think should bring up heartful emotions; however, in reality, they don't. If you find yourself becoming saddened, angered, or frustrated by an image or if you find yourself shifting from image to image, try to settle on an image that brings up authentic heartful states for you. Don't think about it too much. Let the practice guide you. It's the sincere engagement that is most important. Also, remember that some people are not image-based. In other words, just resting in the *felt experience* is sufficient.

Bask in this felt state, while continuing your breathing pattern, as if it were soaking every cell in your body. If your mind wanders, just gently bring it back. Maintain this state for as long as is comfortable, trying to extend the time to twenty minutes if possible.

Practice Sustained HEART at least three times this week and record your experiences in a few paragraphs of narrative. In addition, record brief comments in your practice record log or in your journal. You might entertain some or all of the following questions: How did it feel? Were you able to settle into the practice? What might you change next time? Did you gain any insights from the practice?

Sustained HEART affords many benefits when you practice it regularly: clear thought, fewer worries, a sense of calm or joy, the ability to focus on life without stress intruding. As workshop participant Bryan put it:

> *Immediately, I knew sustained HEART would be beneficial for me. The combination of my workload and outside responsibilities was overwhelming. I had known for a long time that I must do something about this; I was constantly reactive. Sustained HEART kept me sane at a time I should have been quite insane. It is amazing how little time it takes to feel so much better. I ended up feeling calmer and more focused about the rest of my day after every session. I feel like I am becoming a different person.*

The everyday skills of heartful engagement and the practices you are cultivating can be as transformative as your level of engagement with them. Remember, it is helpful to document some of the shifts taking place in your own life. I would suggest that every time you do a HEART practice, you keep up with recording it and your experience with it in your journal.

CONCLUSION: EXPANDING HEART

This chapter led you through a step-by-step process of replacing reactivity with heartful engagement. You have gained an understanding of the diversity of emotional definitions and emotional experience and identified, for yourself, what some heartful emotions are. You have walked through a process to implement them in your day-to-day life through the three-to-one ratio of transformation through emotion. You have learned the importance of authenticity in emotional expression for true transformation, and that intentionality and micromoments are concrete ways you can tip that ratio in your favor. You have identified the opportunities for those moments in your own life. You have reflected and will continue to reflect on the benefits of heartful engagement as they show up for you.

You have been introduced to the power and potential of affect regulation through HEART. You have learned the foundational steps of notice, refocus, and nurture, and you have seen how the practice of HEART can rewire your stress response from emotional chaos to calm and connection. You have practiced regulating your affect in your moments of reactivity, and you have processed what it takes, for you, to set up a sustained practice and begun to make it a regular part of your life.

In the next chapter, you will continue to replace reactivity with specific heartful emotion prescriptions. While this chapter introduced you to the concept of heartful engagement in general, the next builds from that foundation and looks at particular emotions that have been identified in research to directly mitigate some of the difficult emotions that cause and exacerbate stress and anxiety. As you dive deeper in to the application of heartful emotion, you will learn about and implement the antidotes to loneliness through the practice of gratitude. You will first look at what may block you from authentically practicing it and, through a step-by-step process of implementation, experience its transformational power in your own life. Next, you will experience the deep healing powers of empathy and compassion. You will see that they must be experienced for yourself before they can be applied to another, and you will learn a process of rescripting some of the more difficult emotions that surface for you. Lastly, you will be introduced to the power of hope. You will learn what the requirements are for its effective and authentic practice and discover a process to develop it in your own life, leading you to ever greater states of resilience and well-being.

chapter 5

Deepen Your Engagement with Gratitude, Empathy, Compassion, and Hope

In the last chapter, you experienced what heartful emotion feels like for you and gained a deeper understanding of the embodied nature of healing emotion. This further underscored the fact that it is the embodiment of an emotion that most transforms you—good or bad— and to truly rewire a chaotic emotion or problematic stress response, you need to replace it with something entirely different and authentically experienced. The intentional engagement of heartful emotion does this.

This chapter invites a continuation and deepening of both heartful emotion in daily life and HEART by targeting specific emotions. It invites you a step further by engaging in specific emotional prescriptions that have been identified in research to have direct healing potential for some of the reactive states most present in stress and anxiety: loneliness, reactive emotional memory, and hopelessness. You will engage in an authentic practice of gratitude designed to address some of the pitfalls to its effective practice, thus reducing your feelings of loneliness. For example, these pitfalls may include feeling indebted, unworthy, or coerced instead of truly feeling grateful. You will look at some of your deeper reactive patterns in terms of emotional memory, and through self-empathy and compassion, will work to rescript them, and you will learn a step-by-step process to effectively replace a sense of hopelessness with true hope.

The authentic practice of gratitude has been shown to have a myriad of alleviating responses to stress, and reducing feelings of loneliness is one of the most powerful. However, although many positive effects have been documented, there are still great pitfalls to its practice. In this chapter, you will learn about these impediments, how to overcome them, and how to make the practice of gratitude an effective one for you. You will be invited to see the things in your own life you may be grateful for but tend to overlook, you will participate in a new and embodied version of the gratitude journal, and you will practice Everyday Gratitude and Grateful HEART. These are two HEART practices specifically designed to cultivate gratitude in an authentic, routine, and embodied way.

Next, you will experience the deep and healing potential of empathy and compassion for problematic emotions in your life. You will see that you cannot have empathy or compassion for another until you can have them for yourself, and you will understand that they, together, are a necessary two-step process of "holding and healing" through mindful awareness and heartful engagement. Finally, you will implement them for both yourself and others in your life. By revisiting the Emotional Charting exercise from the prior chapter and the emotions below the line, you will identify the emotional states inviting to be rescripted in their implicit patterns of reactivity and learn how to do just that. You will engage in the practice HEART for Holding and Healing Self to cultivate empathy and compassion for yourself, and you will transfer those reflections and practices to others in your life to cultivate a greater sense of understanding and relational healing.

Lastly, you will embody hope. A feeling of hopelessness is often the foundation of stress and a result of it. It is also a state where you normally focus on the all the things you feel are insurmountable and don't see a way beyond your current circumstance. You may think hope as something you *should* have, but it is not tangible; it carries no real vision or promise of something beyond. Research shows that for hope to be a transformative practice, it must include agency, pathways, and visions of a "best possible future self" (Snyder 1989; Peters et al. 2010). These all help you embody a vision of yourself beyond your current struggle. This chapter includes activities and practices, each built from the previous, and designed to cultivate all three of these things. You will recognize your ability for agency through an activity called What Went Well, and Why? You will establish pathways by gaining clarity on what certain things would look like if they *were* working in your life, and you will engage in HEART for Hope, a sustained practice designed to help you embody visions of your best possible future self.

The heartful engagement of gratitude, empathy, compassion, and hope provide a remedy for some of your greatest stress-filled ailments. The order in which these emotions are presented in this chapter is intentional. Gratitude is a stabilizing emotion, and with proper implementation, it is a good entry point for the deeper practice of the emotions that follow.

WHAT GRATITUDE IS—AND HOW IT REDUCES LONELINESS

What is gratitude? What does it have to do with loneliness? You might think gratitude is just the act of being thankful for a specific act from another person. Recently, though, researchers have been generalizing the concept to mean sincere appreciation of anything in the world. However, there are two important elements to this appreciation. The first is that this appreciation carries an affirming of "goodness" in one's life. When you think about, and feel grateful, say, for people who have played pivotal roles in your life, you feel the appreciation throughout your body. And it *feels good* when you recognize this goodness; it truly is a felt, somatic, embodied experience. The second element is that the goodness you feel appreciation for is at least partially outside of the self (Emmons and Stern 2013). And, typically, it is not for the "thing" itself as much as the human experience benefitting from that thing (or person). There is almost always some "connection" factor.

When most people begin to feel grateful for the things in their life, their thoughts almost always expand to the people surrounding those thoughts. And, with the embodied experience of appreciation, these thoughts light up and strengthen the social circuits in their brain. As a result, grateful people, according to research, feel more energetic, alive, enthusiastic, determined, attentive, and alert (Emmons and Crumpler 2000; Emmons and Stern 2013). They feel increased vitality (Wood, Froh, and Geraghty 2010), exercise more regularly, report fewer physically debilitating symptoms of depression (Harbaugh and Vasey 2014) and stress (Wood et al. 2008), and feel better about their life as a whole (Emmons and Stern 2013). Gratitude, by this definition—appreciation for goodness in your life, goodness that comes from outside of you—has been shown to be effective in building on psychological, social, and spiritual resources (Emmons and McCullough 2004). It helps you be more resilient in the face of trauma (Emmons and Stern 2013) and has been shown to reduce cortisol (McCraty et al. 1998), your primary stress hormone; increase oxytocin (Algoe and Way 2014), your primary bonding hormone; and activate parts of your brain associated with social networks (Fox et al. 2015). More often than not, gratitude level is an exceptionally valid predictor of healthy relationships (Algoe, Fredrickson, and Gable 2013).

Thus, the practice of gratitude can change your life. Admittedly, when you are consumed with feelings of loneliness or stress, gratitude feels like an impossible ideal. You may have difficulty seeing beyond the aloneness and dispiritedness that consumes your day. You may feel cut off from those around you and disconnected from life itself. And, from that vantage point, gratitude seems like a pipe dream, an unrealistic notion, or a completely unappealing endeavor. Engagement in a program of gratitude may be the last thing you want to do when you feel consumed with stress and left behind from the deep feelings of attachment that you desire.

As counterintuitive as it seems, a step-by-step approach to cultivating gratitude in your daily life can create a sense of connectedness to the deepest parts of yourself, others, and the outside world. Even when it does not seem like it on the surface, gratitude almost always carries some social connection, and so practicing it—even for the smaller things in your life, ones that don't have to do with other people at all—is a nonthreatening way to approach your connection circuits, or the neural areas in your brain responsible for a sense of personal connectedness (Fox et al. 2015). And the benefits accrue even if your grateful gestures are small. If your current emotional state prevents you from feeling grateful for the bigger things in your life, maybe a walk in the park or appreciating the sunset with a friend will. These smaller shifts "work out" the physiological systems in your body and brain and broaden their capacity for more. The more often you can appreciate the smaller things in your life, the more you are cultivating the capacity for appreciating the larger things.

So, what step-by-step practices can you engage in to promote a heartful and embodied approach to the practice of gratitude? Gratitude is a trainable skill that is available to all. But there are some prerequisites.

UNDERSTAND THE PREREQUISITES FOR GRATITUDE

In terms of heartful engagement, we know that gratitude needs to be authentic, or its embodiment will be decidedly other than a transformational experience. Here is where both the challenge and deep healing potential of gratitude lie. Research has shown that if gratitude expression is done out of a sense of mere indebtedness or ambivalence, the positive effects are mitigated (Chen, Chen, and Tsai 2012; Greenberg and Westcott 1983). In other words, if it is done out of a sense of obligation rather than a sense of true appreciation, the experience will not be a transforming one. For example, you may try to make yourself express gratitude because your religious tradition says you should, or you may keep a perfunctory gratitude list because you have been told it will be good for you, but you do not actually feel authentic gratitude for the things you list. You cannot pretend or force genuine gratitude. In the context of the science of embodiment, this makes perfect sense. The science of embodiment validates that your physiological state and resultant transformational capacities are rooted in your genuine moment-to-moment experience, not in the coerced or ambivalent one. Gratitude training must be authentic, or it is an exercise in futility.

The question is no longer whether gratitude is beneficial or not, but rather how can it be authentically and heartfully cultivated for true healing. And, if you are experiencing feelings of loneliness or isolation, gratitude is both an essential component to personal restoration and a greater challenge to come by. However, even when you feel alienated and isolated from life, if you are able to practice true and authentic gratitude for *something*, the practice can be transforming. In fact, possibly even more so. Research also shows that those with a greater sense of loneliness, isolation, and depression were the ones who benefited the most (Harbaugh and Vasey 2014). The true expression of gratitude is not a superficial Band-Aid with cursory practices that include light engagement. It is a deep, honest, and heartful engagement with those things in your life for which you are most grateful. The more deeply and heartfully you engage, the more transformation you will experience.

Following is a step-by-step process comprising written exercises, activities, and contemplative practices designed to reduce your feelings of isolation and loneliness through the intentional, authentic, and heartful engagement of gratitude. Given the requirement of authenticity, I encourage you to do these exercises with an ever-present awareness of the truth of your experience. If it feels coerced or if feelings of guilt, ambivalence, inadequacy, or indebtedness begin to surface, hold these feelings in self-compassionate, nonjudgmental awareness and progress in a way that feels comfortable and true for you. Those are all common experiences, are the biggest impediments to cultivating true gratitude, and are exceptionally important to acknowledge from a place of self-understanding and self-compassion. There are no "shoulds" in gratitude.

You will be invited to, from an experiential place, look for the good things in your life that you literally might not see because your focus is on all your challenges, to bring a deeper and consistent awareness to the things in your life for which you are grateful, and to learn practices to more deeply cultivate gratitude in your life.

A HEARTFUL PRESCRIPTION FOR GRATITUDE

This heartful prescription for gratitude contains three steps:

1. Identify your "gorillas."

2. Keep the prescribed version of a gratitude journal.

3. Practice Everyday Gratitude and Grateful HEART.

Identify Your Gorillas

The practice and development of gratitude invites you to see what may be elusive in your typical awareness. You cannot be grateful for things you do not "see." However, if you are like most people, you go through a good portion of your day consumed with an inner dialogue that is primarily narrating a life of challenge. It may be telling you that you are not good enough and everything is stacked against you. What is more, you may have unknowingly trained yourself to only see or per-ceive those things in your life that match that dialogue, completely missing the life-sustaining things that are ever-present and, for the most part, overlooked. One of the first aspects of cultivating gratitude is training yourself to see that to which you might ordinarily be blind.

The concept of "selective attention" or "in-attentional blindness" explains that you are blind to the things that you do not pay attention to, and the things that you do pay attention to will show up for you full force. One of the most famous demonstrations of this was an experi-ment in which individuals were shown a video of people, some in white shirts and some in black, passing basketballs to each other, and instructed to watch for players in white shirts throwing to other players in white. Seventy-nine percent of those who watched this video were so consumed by this task that they didn't even notice that there was a person in a gorilla costume who walked to the middle of the group and pounded its chest before continuing on (Neisser and Hyman 1982). When you are hyperfocused on one thing, you may miss other things that are literally right in front of your face. Research has shown over and over again that you perceive only those objects that receive your focused attention (Hillyard and Anllo-Vento 1998).

Selective attention plays itself out over and over again in your daily life. Further, you only have the capacity for so much conscious awareness. In other words, your brain can only pay attention to so much at once, so if you are giving the things in your life that are challenging more emotional attention than they deserve, you may completely miss the good things that are right in front of your face. And neuroscience confirms that what you pay attention to wires you to see more of the same. So, when you are focused on what you think is wrong; what may go wrong; or what could, should, or would go wrong, you not only miss seeing the wonderful things right in front of you, but quite often you miss the opportunity to cultivate more of their presence. Paying attention to the gorillas that surround you—the daily graces you tend to overlook or not see at all—can profoundly change the way you see the world.

Exercise and Reflection: What Are Your Gorillas?

In this exercise, the term "gorilla" represents the good things in your life you may overlook or not routinely "see" in their full presence. What graces in your life are you overlooking? What are your gorillas? Write and brainstorm about the wonderful things in your life you may be overlooking because your awareness is directed at your many challenges. Write in a stream-of-consciousness style, and let the writing lead you. What are you overlooking? What might be different if you gave it more of your heartful engagement?

"The gorilla was my girlfriend" was the opening line of a thank-you letter I received from Jon. Here is his story.

Jon was in a four-year relationship that was rapidly deteriorating because he was so focused on his own stresses from work and school that he was taking for granted the presence of his girlfriend. He used to make time to nurture their relationship, but he had been overlooking what he had originally appreciated in her: her kindness, her support of him, and the fact that they shared so many mutual interests. Instead of making time for their relationship, he had recently become so preoccupied with work that he was either not physically or emotionally present because, when he was there, he would just zone out in front of the television.

When she tried to talk to him about it, he just perceived her as nagging and not understanding his stress. Instead of looking forward to the marriage they had planned on, they were now thinking of splitting up. All he could see in his relationship were the problems his fiancé, and their relationship, posed in his life, and he was seriously questioning if it was working.

After watching the in-attentional blindness video, he was shocked he had missed the gorilla. When he engaged in the What Are Your Gorillas? exercise, he realized his girlfriend had become his gorilla. He had completely lost sight of all the beauty and happiness she had brought into his life. He realized that because he was so focused on his stress, he had completely lost sight of the appreciation he had for her and the qualities he originally fell in love with.

This realization led to substantial changes that saved their struggling relationship. When he realized that he was no longer "seeing" his girlfriend, he began to make small shifts to see her in a new light, even just asking her to watch something they both enjoyed on TV. He also began to build in intentional time to nurture their relationship in the way he did when they were first dating. The small moments of seeing her "new again" completely transformed their relationship from one of struggle to one that was flourishing. The spiral of their connection became one of newness and rebirth, and he reported that he felt like he was falling in love all over again. And it was all by choice of gratitude through attention.

"Seeing new" and keeping a gratitude journal can help you begin to identify things in your life for which you are grateful, and it can prepare you for the deeper gratitude practices to follow. Simply put, it is an effective "entryway" to begin a more involved practice of gratitude. However, it needs authentic engagement, not perfunctory adherence.

Journal About Gratitude

Many practices of gratitude engage in writing gratitude lists, keeping a gratitude jar, or writing a gratitude journal. And the research on these practices has been overwhelmingly positive, especially in the reduction of feelings of isolation and loneliness. However, if it is done perfunctorily, superficially, or without regard to the authentic emotion being experienced, the beneficial effects are marginal at best and may even be counterproductive. If it is not an authentic experience or expression, it is not truly gratitude. Further, if the other feelings are dominant, like feeling compelled to *have* to write a list, those are the ones to which you are adapting. Gratitude cannot be faked, it cannot be forced, and it cannot be coerced. Further, if you are overcome with guilt or debilitating feelings of unworthiness in its pursuit, you are experiencing and adapting to something decidedly different.

Recall that the science of embodiment demonstrates that for an experience to truly be transformative, it must be felt deeply enough to be exhibited in our physiological systems of adaptation. Merely going through perfunctory motions without the truth of experience is not sufficient. Starting, intending to feel gratitude, and feeling something else is counterproductive. The following exercise is an extension of the popular gratitude list or journal; however, it invites you into a deeper experience of gratitude's felt occurrence. Remember, for any heartful experience to be transformative, it needs to be truly felt. It is better to focus on fewer, truer experiences than many ambivalent ones.

Exercise and Reflection: The Gratitude Journal

For the next four days, pick one to three things in your life to journal about. Rather than listing many, the idea of this activity is to authentically engage with fewer, at a deeper level. Aim to write for about twenty minutes and focus on what it is about your objects of gratitude that you are truly thankful for. Focus on the details that bring up the felt response of gratitude and be especially aware if other contradictory feelings surface, such as guilt, unworthiness, or distressing indebtedness. If any other feelings surface, notice without judgment and switch to something else that you can experience authentically.

Variation. Write a letter of gratitude to someone to whom you are grateful. They can be living or deceased, and the letter does not have to be delivered (although research has shown a powerful effect, if they are still living, when the letter or message is delivered in person [Seligman 2011]). The idea is to write descriptively enough to elicit a felt response within you as you bring your awareness to the recognition of your gratitude for the other.

Once you have trained yourself to begin to authentically focus on gratitude and notice where it might play out in your life, it is time to focus on a more deliberate practice of the embodied state of gratitude.

Grateful Practices

An important component of this prescription for gratitude development is the associated practices, both Grateful HEART and Everyday Gratitude. Everyday Gratitude focuses on noticing, pausing, and really soaking up the embodied state of gratitude as the opportunities present themselves throughout the day, and Grateful HEART is a sustained practice of gratitude where you intentionally and deeply experience states of gratitude in a designated contemplative practice. Both build on the skills you have cultivated through the last activities. Consistent use of these practices creates the time and depth of experience necessary for substantial change at the physiological, or embodied, level. An exceedingly important point to notice, however, is the possible emergence of feelings other than gratitude. If feelings other than genuine gratitude arise, acknowledge them and shift your focus to something or someone for whom you can feel authentic gratitude.

Practice: Everyday Gratitude

When you bring conscious awareness to any moment and focus on the felt experience of that moment, you bring an embodied awareness that helps you store it as such. In other words, hyperfocusing on moments of your life, as if you were trying to make a physiological imprint of those moments right in that moment, actually helps to do just that. The practice of Everyday Gratitude takes merely noticing moments of gratitude one step further. It invites you to pause, reflect, and intentionally soak up the *felt experience* of that moment. This practice not only deepens the physiological experience of the moment, creating shifts in your temporary point of view, it also creates long-term foundational changes in your embodied capacities for gratitude. When you have identified a moment for which to be grateful, soak up that felt experience as if you were trying to cement the memory in your cells. Sustain this felt experience as long as is comfortable and appropriate for the situation.

Practice: Grateful HEART

Grateful HEART is an extension of the other HEART practices in that it is built on the steps of notice, refocus, and nurture—with the nurture step, in this case, centering on the heartful experience of gratitude for the things in your life you can really embody or have a sustained *felt sense* of gratitude toward. Again, it is built from the Sustained HEART practice, and you may want to reread the longer description (in chapter 5). A shorter description follows. For a recording of these instructions, go to http://www.newharbinger.com/42839.

1. *Notice:* Notice your thoughts, your emotions, and your bodily sensations and disengage from them, or witness them, without judgment.

2. *Refocus:* Release all the tension—in the muscles around your eyes, in the muscles of your shoulders, anywhere in the body it might be. Let your awareness drop to a place in your torso that feels comfortable for you. Focus on slow, natural, comfortable breaths at that focal point.

3. *Nurture:* Hold a person or several people for whom you are authentically grateful in your awareness. You do not need to feel gratitude for a specific thing or act, but rather, you are focusing on a general sense of appreciation. Let the practice lead you. In other words, do not think too hard about trying to figure out whom to focus on; let the images or sensations come to you as if you were scrolling through various aspects of your life and letting certain people emerge. Hold these people in a felt sense of appreciation and notice what is about the role they have played in your life that you are grateful for. Try to rest in a deep sensation of gratitude for ten to fifteen minutes.

Notice through subsequent days whether more people appear in your awareness during the practice and throughout the day.

Maintenance. Spend at least ten minutes every day on your gratitude journal. Practice Everyday Gratitude in all the moments it feels comfortable to do so and practice Grateful HEART at least once a week.

The authentic cultivation of gratitude can change your life, almost in direct proportion to how deeply you are able to engage in its practice. It is a deeper and more specific application of the heartful engagement introduced in the last chapter. It also provides a foundation of stability necessary for the next practices. The next specific prescriptions to heartful emotion—those for self-empathy and compassion—invite you into a deeper application, and it is important to approach these exercises after you have incorporated the general ideas of heartful engagement and gratitude first. In essence, they require a little more heartful "muscle"—the muscle you have developed from the previous practices. The exercises and practices for empathy and compassion are designed to address problematic implicit memory patterns that may be coloring your perceptions—those that you might sometimes feel hijacked by because they are fueled by an emotion you wrote below the line on the chart.

Many popular approaches to stress management and emotional healing will label these all-consuming emotions as "negative" or "afflictive" and deem them as things to be overcome or judged because they are inherently bad. You may have been taught, or led to believe, that these emotions are not, nor should, be welcomed and the only way to deal with them is to overpower them, suppress them, or pretend you are not feeling them. I rarely characterize those above the line as positive and those below the line as negative because that assumes an inherent judgment of what we might term as negative.

A heartfully engaged approach to difficult emotion invites you into a radically different way of being with or healing these states; it also invites you past the debilitating self-blame, shame, judgment, and feelings of worthlessness that typically surround them. I often say, "Shift when you can; heal when you can't." The cultivation of empathy and compassion, as represented here, is a powerful path to that healing and counteract the more individual problematic emotions that may be troubling you.

CULTIVATE EMPATHY AND COMPASSION

This section invites you into deep states of healing, for yourself and your relationships, through the cultivation of empathy and compassion. This path to fostering empathy and compassion requires that you first develop them for yourself, for you cannot effectively feel them for another if you are immersed in your own emotional chaos. This process is directed inward and proposes a fundamental "holding and healing" of that which is difficult. Once you have developed them for yourself, you then learn to "hold and heal" the relationships in your life.

> *Kendra hated herself for not being able to be there for her grandmother. Her grandmother was aging, had taken ill, and wanted Kendra to come by twice a week to cook for her when the visiting nurse could not be there. All at once, Kendra felt blamed and judged by her grandmother for her resistance, angry that she was even being asked because she was so overwhelmed with her other responsibilities, and ashamed of herself for feeling all those things. What was the big deal? Clearly there was something else going on.*

UNDERSTAND AND DISTINGUISH EMPATHY AND COMPASSION

While empathy and compassion are certainly related, and often confused or used interchangeably, it is important to understand their distinctions for the practices that follow.

Empathy is most often defined as "the sharing and understanding of another's experience" (Ashar et al. 2016). The prefix "em" means "go into," and in the case of empathy, it can be understood as going "into" another's experience and thus gaining a deep understanding of that experience. Further, in the form of self-empathy, the "other" is you. From an imaginative space, you will be deeply "witnessing" your own story.

It is also very important to note that empathy can become its own form of distress if two considerations are not present. First, there must be "perspective taking" on the part of the empathizer (Leiberg and Anders 2006; Ruby and Decety 2004). In other words, there needs to be a differentiation between self and other. If there is no differentiation, the empathizer absorbs the distress of the person to which they are feeling empathy. From an embodied perspective, this makes total sense: if I make another's experience mine, I suffer all the associated physiological outcomes.

In the form of self-empathy, this is the nonreactive, nonjudgmental full "witnessing" of mindful awareness. You are fully aware and witnessing your own story, but from the point of view of an observer. Through a written activity and deep contemplative practice, you will "hold" your own story as if you were another, witnessing your story in deep yet emotionally grounded understanding.

The second necessary component to prevent empathy from becoming its own form of distress is that it be followed by compassion. That is the shift to heartful engagement. Compassion is often defined as the prosocial behavior of being with another in their suffering (Ashar et al. 2016; Singer and Kilmecki 2014) and motivated to help heal it. So, while they are surely associated, there seems to be consensus that compassion takes empathy a step further by not only understanding and witnessing but by being moved to relieve associated pain around experience.

Through writing and deep contemplative practice, you will imaginatively "heal" your implicit memories by providing what that memory needs to become emotionally balanced. In other words, through self-compassionate imagery, you will offer a new experience for your neural nets to replace the old experience. One of my favorite examples of how this self-compassionate imagery works is in a story of the magical tricycle that Louis Cozolino shares (Cozolino 2010) in his book *The Neuroscience of Psychotherapy*. He tells the story of a man who was a child in the holocaust. Every time the man would feel the resurfacing anxiety from his past memories, he would deeply imagine himself as a child, but then change the memory by imagining and deeply feeling the experience of a magic tricycle coming down from the sky and taking him away to a place of magic and beauty.

Before you learn the process of "holding and healing" and read about Kendra's experience as she went through this process, let us review both your emotional charting exercise and the workings of implicit memory, as these are what this process aims to heal and rebalance.

CULTIVATE EMPATHY AND COMPASSION FOR YOURSELF

The exercises of self-empathy and self-compassion in this section ask you to revisit the Emotional Charting exercise you completed in the last chapter as well as the concepts of implicit memory presented in chapter 1. When you did the Emotional Charting exercise, you were asked to brainstorm your life-generating emotional states and list them above the line and to brainstorm your life-degenerative emotional states and list them below the line. Further, recall from the spiral of becoming that your perceptions and reactions are filtered from what is stored in your implicit memory, or past experience. Implicit memory and the emotional states below the line are profoundly connected.

Recall that through implicit memory, when you have had difficult experiences, as we have all had to some degree or another, those experiences are stored to help you make meaning of future circumstance. They color the lens of the things you interpret and tell you how to feel and think. If you have experienced difficult emotion before, such as neglect, shame, or judgment, and some current circumstance "looks" similar (possibly remotely), you will place the old meaning on the new circumstance and see everything through that lens. Further, you adopt behaviors and choices from your continued perceptions through these emotions. *They can hijack your whole emotional system and are most likely the states you wrote below the line on the chart.* These are typically learned responses from the memory itself, the pain it caused, or behaviors you have adapted to shield yourself from like occurrences.

When you are hijacked by one of these emotional states, you might let it consume you, you might try to suppress it, or you might blame, shame, or judge yourself for having it. None of those work, and you experience them all the more. They are contrary to any physiological state of healing.

How, then, do you heal? You heal by going to the source. You heal by creating new experience, and, properly applied, practices of self-empathy and self-compassion can provide that experience through contemplative practice. Simply put, through a combination of meditation and imagination, you are giving your neural networks new experiences that take the emotional charge out of problematic implicit memories, or those states below the line.

CREATE NEW NEURAL CONNECTIONS BY "HOLDING AND HEALING"

Though past stress and distress are wired in your neural networks and implicit memory, your brain and body are not static; they are constantly forming to experience. And new experience can interrupt that old wiring by encouraging the development of new, healthy neural connections instead. What's more, this can be done through imagined experience as well as actual experience, as your brain doesn't know the difference between what is vividly imagined and what is true. In other words, the rewiring of the implicit memory can be done through contemplative practice by deeply engaging in an imagined experience.

This process has been referred to as memory rescripting, imagery rescripting, or, more recently, memory reconsolidation, and has been shown to be effective in a multitude of circumstances (Agren 2014). Its practice has the capacity to fundamentally alter or erase emotional memory without disrupting the associated autobiographical memory (Agren 2014). In other words, you can still remember the event, but the emotional charge around it and its impact on your future perceptions are lessened or erased altogether. Simply put, through imagery, you rewire the emotional impact of past events and clear the lens for your present and future.

It is also important to note that the memory you are recalling does not have to be a factual one. In other words, if the memory is too intense, or beyond conscious awareness, a representative image will work. You need only access the neural nets enough to "unlock" them, and this can be done through any image or feeling that brings up for you the associated emotion. Memory reconsolidation is built on three components. First, you unlock the associated neural networks of the memory just enough to access them. Second, you destabilize them by not offering the same emotional response you usually do, and third, you offer a mismatch in experience (Ecker 2015; Agren 2014).

As it is offered here, it is a two-step process. The first step consists of bringing to mind an emotional memory and breaking the old patterns by not responding in your typical ways; you hold the memory, and response, in a witnessing, disengaged, nonreactive state of self-empathy. The second step is to be with those implicit patterns from a place of self-compassion with a desire to heal them and, through your imagination, to offer a mismatch or healing experience. This is the process of "holding and healing."

When you can first hold these states, even as reactive, uncomfortable, or painful as they are now, in a place of understanding and nonjudgmental, nonreactive, full presence, you begin to cultivate a physiological state of healing by unlocking the associated neural nets and destabilizing their structure. Instead of reacting in your typical ways, you can witness and form an empathetic awareness of them as you would a best friend. This is the healing power of self-empathy. You hold your difficult emotion in a mindful presence without reactivity and without judgment, and this "witnessing" begins to heal you. It heals by both changing your typical response patterns, thus breaking those familiar neural connections, and creating a new experience of "being seen." This nonreactivity and empathetic witnessing can be an exercise in itself; however, it is also a prerequisite to the active and intentional engagement of self-compassion.

After "holding" your difficult emotions with empathetic nonreactivity, self-compassion invites an active and intentional engagement of being with them in a whole new way. Through self-compassionate imagery, you are offering a mismatch of the old experience and replacing—or reconsolidating—those memories with a new emotional experience. In other words, instead of suppressing it or taking off with the reaction, you bring it to mind, hold it in a nonjudgmental witnessing, and then offer an alternative imagined experience and loving connection to that piece of you that is experiencing the emotion—almost like you would a best friend. The process offered here has been heavily influenced by the work of Richard Schwartz and Frank Rogers (Schwartz 1997; Rogers 2015).

Through this heartful connection, even to your past difficult experience, you are rewiring the neural networks of your implicit memory. You don't lose the conscious memory, but you reform the chaotic emotion that accompanies it and reduce its impact on all your future perceptions.

Although the following exercises are designed to be done back-to-back, it is important to give each your full attention. Doing so leads you through the necessary process of fully witnessing (unlocking and destabilizing) before being moved to heal (offering a mismatch from the old experience).

When Kendra reflected on her Emotional Charting exercise, the words that immediately jumped out at her were "anger," "shame," and "abandonment"; the word "abandonment" surprised her. She imagined herself as a "best friend" telling her story, and, when writing, the words just began to flow. As she listened, she realized the anger and shame were responses directed at her grandmother to cover up the deeper feelings of abandonment that somehow were surfacing. The feelings of abandonment stemmed from her mother and had nothing to do with her grandmother. She continued to just fully witness a third-person version of herself telling her full story.

Exercise and Reflection: Cultivate Self-Empathy

Turn back to the emotional charting exercise you did in the last chapter. Look at the difficult emotional states that you wrote below the line. Pick one that you would like to work on. See if you can disengage from any emotional reaction you might have as you entertain the difficult feeling. If you cannot, if it is too powerful, pick another one that you can work on first. After you have disengaged from any reactivity, imagine a best friend experiencing the difficult feeling. From a nonreactive, nonjudgmental stance, write, in a stream-of-consciousness style, why your friend may experience that difficult emotion. Do not try to "figure it out" as much as just hold and understand your friend's experience. You might even write, in the third person, from the standpoint of your friend, why they feel that way. Notice if any images come up for you. They may be images of you in the past or related past memories. Remember, it is crucially important that you do this from a nonreactive, nonjudgmental, "observing" or "witnessing" point of view, maybe even with a little curiosity or surprise. You might simply ask your friend, "What is your story?"

Exercise and Reflection: Cultivate Self-Compassion

Extending now the Cultivate Self-Empathy exercise, reengage with the image of the best friend experiencing the difficult emotion. Write, from a stream-of-consciousness style, what you would perceive that best friend needs for healing. And, remember, it is important to write from a third-person point of view, as if it were a best friend, possibly even a twin or a somewhat removed sense of yourself. It is also important to let "them" tell you what they need, not try to figure it out from a cognitive, first-person point of view.

It is fundamentally important to remember, however, that when working with memory rescripting, the "need" is often not in present time. In other words, it may involve what you needed in a past scenario that you didn't get; this imagery is what recodes the problematic implicit memory. Further, it doesn't have to be grounded in reality. Like the man with the magic tricycle, what he needed was merely an image he could give to his "child" to heal his emotional memory. Be creative in what imagery works for you.

Let the writing lead you. Sufficient space and time for "them" to really be able to express what they need is important in this exercise. Also of importance is that you receive this information from a nonjudgmental and nonreactive full presence. You might simply ask your "friend," "What do you need?"

After Kendra let her "friend" fully tell her story, she realized that when her parents split up, she felt very abandoned by her mother and that that young girl in her needed to be loved. In the following HEART practice, she deeply imagined herself getting the love and nurturing she didn't get then.

Practice: HEART for Holding and Healing Self

Remember, in all the HEART practices, the notice and refocus steps are the same. The nurture step in HEART for Holding and Healing is to first let your "best friend" or "twin" share with you why they feel the way they do when they experience this difficult emotion. Don't try to figure it out too much; just let the meditation guide you. Let it organically unfold with your "friend" sharing their experience. Your job is just to hold them and witness their story from an empathic yet nonreactive presence. Second, after giving sufficient time for fully witnessing their story, let them tell you what they need now or needed then—it may include both. To listen to a recording of this practice, go to http://www.newharbinger.com/42839.

1. *Notice* your reactivity in your thoughts, emotions, and bodily responses and disengage from it, or witness it.

2. *Refocus* your physiological response by releasing the muscles in your eyes and shoulders, dropping your attention to your torso, and establishing a grounded breathing pattern.

3. *Nurture:* Once you are deep into the meditative state, revisit the Cultivate Self-Empathy exercise. Give yourself sufficient time to resettle in to a place of nonjudgment and full listening. This should take several minutes to fully engage with your "best friend," how they experience this difficult emotion, and any story behind it. After you have settled into the "holding" place of deep empathy, begin to envelop this image in a healing presence by extending loving compassion. Next, deeply imagine giving them what they need or needed at another time and didn't get. It is also important that it be a *felt experience* of extending love and compassion, and also of receiving it, as the felt experience is what creates the physiological changes necessary for true healing. In this practice, you are at once both the giver and receiver of deep compassionate feelings. Hold this deep connection for approximately ten minutes, or as long as is comfortable.

It is often helpful to journal after the practice, as additional and important insights may come up.

After the practice, Kendra realized that her feelings of abandonment, repressed from her mother, were now being transferred to her grandmother. She realized that she was afraid of her grandmother leaving like her mother did. When she had this realization, her anger and shame diminished, and it freed her up to be simply present with her grandmother.

CULTIVATE EMPATHY AND COMPASSION FOR ANOTHER

A fundamentally important insight in being able to affectively develop empathy and compassion for others is to realize that they, just as you, are controlled by the implicit memory patterns that have been programmed into their psyche since day one. Just as you have difficult implicit memories that cause you to have feelings or exhibit behaviors that are not really "you" at your core, so do they. Unless they are in a calm and grounded state, what you see and experience as their external behavior is likely a composite of their implicit memory patterns and learned behaviors. And the more extreme their demeanor, the more likely their implicit programming is in charge. These exercises and practices invite you to look beyond another's implicit programming and learned behaviors, and witness and "be with" the core of who they are.

Exercise and Reflection:
Empathy for Another

Pick someone for whom you would like to develop empathy and compassion. Turn back to the Emotional Charting exercise in the last chapter. Create an emotional chart for them as you think they would experience it. Once you have completed the chart, pick a difficult emotion at the bottom of the chart that you would more fully like to understand how they experience. Write, as if they were telling you their story from their point of view, why and how they experience this emotion. As you write, imagine you are listening to their story, and write in a stream-of-consciousness style from a nonjudgmental point of view. Just witness and hold their story. It is important to note that you don't need to know their complete factual story. Just intuitively let your writing lead you to what you think their emotional experience might be. Also, notice any reactivity that may come up in you. Hold your responses as well in a nonjudgmental and witnessing stance.

Exercise and Reflection:
Compassion for Another

Extending now the Empathy for Another exercise, re-engage in your mind with the person for whom you would like to develop compassion. Write, from a stream-of-consciousness style, what you would perceive them to need for healing as they are experiencing this difficult emotion. It is also important to let them tell you what they need and not try to figure it out from a cognitive, first-person point of view. Again, you are writing as if they are telling you, and you are able to receive this information from a full and loving presence. Let the writing lead you. Sufficient space and time to nonjudgmentally listen to them authentically express what they need is important in this exercise. Also of importance is that you receive this information from a nonjudgmental point of view and be aware of any reactions you may be experiencing that block you from being able to be with this information in a loving and compassionate way.

When Kendra did the following exercise to try to understand her grandmother's behavior, she realized that she (Kendra's grandmother), too, had tender implicit memories around the dynamics with her daughter—Kendra's mother. She realized the insistent pressuring around wanting Kendra to be there was also caused by the past hurt of her daughter, the fear and sadness of losing her, too, and Kendra was able to see the situation, and her grandmother, in a new light.

Practice: HEART for Holding and Healing Another

After performing the notice and refocus steps of the standard HEART protocol, this practice invites you to engage in an empathetic and compassionate encounter with another. Your job is just to contemplatively hold them and witness their story from an empathic yet nonreactive presence. Second, after giving sufficient time for fully witnessing their story, let them tell you what they need now or needed then—the response may include both. To listen to a recording of this practice, go to http://www.newharbinger.com/42839.

1. *Notice* your reactivity in your thoughts, emotions, and bodily responses and disengage from it, or witness it.

2. *Refocus* your physiological response by releasing the muscles in your eyes and shoulders, dropping your attention to your torso, and establishing a grounded breathing pattern.

3. *Nurture:* Once you are deep into the meditative state, revisit the empathetic understanding for another you gained in the associated exercise, and imagine yourself "holding" the other's experience in a state of full empathy. Give yourself sufficient time to settle in to a place of full listening; this should take several minutes to fully re-engage with the previous exercise. After you have settled again into the holding place of deep empathy, begin to be with this person by extending loving compassion. If it feels comfortable to do so, imagine yourself giving to them what they expressed they needed in the previous exercise. It is important to imagine the "core" of you extending this love and compassion to the "core" of them. It is also important that it be a *felt experience.* Hold this deep connection for approximately ten minutes, or as long as is comfortable.

Supplemental activity. This is an extremely rich time to journal. If it feels comfortable to do so, journal about your experience with the practice and notice any additional insights.

After engaging in the above practices, it is important to reflect on your experience. What did it feel like? Were you able to fully engage? What insights did you gain?

Maintenance. Practice HEART for Holding and Healing Self and HEART for Holding and Healing Another as often as you are called. If it feels comfortable, do so at least twice a week. Also, when you are working on self-empathy and self-compassion, you might continue to work with other emotions below the line for continued emotional balance and healing. You can make these practices an ongoing part of your practice repertoire for continual growth and resilience from reactive patterns.

Empathy and compassion, properly applied, can be profoundly healing; they allow you to hold the experiences of others in a whole new light. Further, they are healing for you as well. They have been shown to significantly improve many of the debilitating states associated with stress.

Compassion has been shown to engage your physiological systems and brain areas most closely associated with connection and calm, decreasing negative affect and increasing positive affect (Klimecki et al. 2013, 2014). In other words, it not only reduces the negative, it creates the positive. Its practice has been shown to increase positive emotions, improve physical health, reduce your stress response (Ashar et al. 2016), and increase oxytocin, the bonding and connecting hormone (Bos et al. 2015). Cultivating compassion creates and strengthens prosocial patterns in your brain (Ashar et al. 2016), enhances brain areas involved in emotional processing and empathy, and enhances your immune response (Hofmann, Grossman, and Hinton 2011). It has been associated with increasing personal resources such as purpose in life and social support and increasing the overall impact of positive emotions in one's life (Fredrickson et al. 2008). A compassionate attitude or stance has been shown to modulate the activity of the amygdala, or calm the emotional processing center of your brain (Kim et al. 2009). More simply, compassion training helps you feel better about your life, feel a deeper connection with others, feel less stress, improve your health, get sick less often, feel emotionally calmer, understand your emotions better, and be more socially motivated to help others.

Properly practiced, empathy and compassion lead you ever more up the continuum of emotional integration and further your capacities to more fully live from a dominant calm and connection system.

Healing through empathy and compassion, for both self and other, also leads you to new spaces for hope to open up. But what is true hope? And how is it effectively cultivated?

CULTIVATE HOPE

Sometimes the concept of hope may feel like a disdained ideal or an empty wish. Hope, for many people, often feels like a vague construct or lofty ideal that has no constructive use in everyday reality. Worse, the idea of it may just exacerbate the divide between what you perceive as your current circumstance and what you wish were true. You may feel that the concept of hope basically asks you to put your faith in something you really do not believe or don't think you can achieve; so, what good is it?

However, this is an inaccurate interpretation of hope. Hope is not merely wishing for something different; rather, it is a better sense of the future, a sense of confidence in it. And this is a confidence you can cultivate—even if it doesn't feel like it at the moment.

Research has shown that the intentional development of hope has a resilience effect that counteracts feelings of hopelessness (Huen et al. 2015) and produces feelings of overall resilience and optimism (Huen et al. 2015). Research also shows that there are some very specific processes for the effective development of hope. These have been identified as developing "agency and pathways" (Snyder 1989) and a vision of your "best possible future self" (Peters et al. 2010). These are actual steps you can take to transform the idea of hope from an empty wish to a confident outlook for the future. And the activities and practices in this section are designed to help you take them.

This section invites you into a heartfully engaged interpretation of hope through a step-by-step process to effectively cultivate it in your own life. It offers you the opportunity to create confidence in your future by identifying and appreciating your own agency, gaining clarity on what it is you do want, and lovingly connect with your best possible future self.

A HEARTFUL PRESCRIPTION FOR HOPE

This heartful prescription for hope contains three steps:

1. *Realize your agency* by reflecting on "What went well, and why?"

2. *Gain hope by establishing clarity* on what you do want.

3. *Visualize and connect with* your future self.

These three steps are designed to help you develop the agency and pathways necessary for the cultivation of true hope. When you see that you have the internal resources, or more capacity to invoke change than you might have previously thought, and can *authentically* see and lovingly connect with a vision of yourself beyond your current circumstance, hope begins to replace hopelessness, and you act accordingly.

REALIZE YOUR AGENCY

Though it may be hard to remember this when stress is really strong, there are likely things that are actually going well in your life. And you most likely have some agency in the things that are going well. In other words, when you do recall those things, you may think they have nothing to do with *you*, but this may not be the case. The following exercise is designed to focus your attention on the things that are going well in your life—and your role in making those good things happen.

Exercise and Reflection: What Went Well, and Why?

This exercise is inspired by Martin Seligman (Seligman 2013). The invitation of the exercise is to identify at least three things during your day that went well and describe why you think they went well.

Draw a line down the middle of a piece of paper. On the left-hand side, write at the top "What went well?" and title the right-hand side "Why?" For example, on the left side, you might write that you and your partner got along well after work, and on the right side, you might write that you were fully present in the conversation you shared about your respective days. Or, on the right side, you might write that a project at work went well, and on the left side acknowledge that you were prepared when working on it. *Focus on your contribution* to what you noted went well and let yourself appreciate the impact of your agency—or the hand you played in it going well. The list does not need to comprise major things in your day if that does not feel authentic. Small but sincere things will do fine.

What did you learn? What roles do you or did you play in the things that are actually going right for you? Can you identify some of your personal strengths through this process?

Beyond focusing on your own agency, true hope requires a "vision beyond." If you are like most people, when you are feeling lost or hopeless about a specific circumstance in your life or life in general, you are so focused on what you *do not* want that you don't really have a sense of what you *do* want. You just know you want things to be different. Although you may have a vague idea, you likely have no concrete grasp or image of what it would truly "look like" if it were working. If cultivating hope is developing confidence in a better future, gaining clarity on what that future circumstance would look like is an important step on the path.

GAIN HOPE BY ESTABLISHING CLARITY

Clarity fosters hope and helps you realize your "pathways." Remember, your brain has a limited capacity for awareness. Bringing full, clear, and specific awareness to all the areas in your life in which you would like to cultivate and developing a sense of clarity brings a sense of hope, or an ability to see beyond what may be currently troubling you. Exercises in clarity also show that when you can bring your awareness to the things you do want in your life, you are more likely to work to manifest them. And, when you bring deep detail to a problem and how it might be solved, the answers of how to get there automatically emerge (Senge, Schwarmer, and Flowers 2004). The more specific you are about the details, the more your attention is focused on the "answer" instead of the problem.

Next, is a writing activity designed to help you develop clarity and a loving connection to a vision of yourself beyond your struggles. It is loosely based on the work of Michael Losier (Losier 2007).

Exercise and Reflection: Discern Clarity

In this exercise, you will write a specific, detailed description of the aspects of a situation in your life in which you would like to see change. Draw a line down the middle of a page. On the left side, write in depth about the specifics of the situation that are not working. Pay attention to detail. This is not meant to be an exercise in which you immerse yourself in a sense of hopelessness as much as a mindful and observational approach to discerning, from a disengaged point of view, exactly what is not working. On the right hand of the paper, write, also in depth and with detail, what the situation would "look" like if it were working. Heartfully engage and get as clear as you can about the vision and detail of how the improved situation would appear in your life.

You can write narratively or write a bulleted list, but the greater the detail, the more the potential for hope. An important aspect of this exercise is that you do not have to figure out the means whereby or how to get there yet. First, you only bring awareness to what it would look like if it were working. The more in depth you can write about the detail of the problem and what it would look like if it were truly working, the more likely the answers of the means to get there will automatically emerge.

Add-on exercise. If, when you were completing the above exercise, steps you can take to implement change began to appear, address them in a stream-of-consciousness style.

What did you learn? How has clarity shed new light on your issue? Process and reflect in a way that is comfortable for you.

VISUALIZE AND CONNECT WITH YOUR FUTURE SELF

Hope invites you to feel confident about the future and rest in the felt experience of that confident vision. In the last exercise, you gained some specific clarity on how parts of your life might look if they were flourishing. Now you will take your journey to hope a step further. As you have learned, from an embodied perspective, the more you experience anything, the better you get at making that experience your reality. Further, important parts of your brain do not know the difference between what is vividly imagined and what is real—and will adapt accordingly. Research has shown that imagery activates and changes the perceptual centers of the brain (Cichy, Heinzle, and Haynes 2012). In other words, vividly imagining a scenario impacts the deep parts of the brain that perceive and then create a corresponding outcome. The rest of the HEART practices rely heavily on imagery to rewire you to resilience and well-being.

Practice: HEART for Hope

HEART for Hope invites you to take what you learned in the previous exercise for clarity and create an image of yourself flourishing in those areas you wrote about. In this practice, you will hold an image of yourself already beyond the struggle. Pay attention to specific details in the practice and let yourself *feel* the experience. Again, feelings around this image must be authentic. If negative thoughts, feelings, or doubts surface, switch to an image to which you can feel a hopeful connection. If an image is hard for you to authentically feel, start slowly with an image in your past where you felt something similar—it can be as simple as learning to tie your shoes—and work your way up. To listen to a recording of this practice, go to http://www.newharbinger .com/42839.

1. *Notice* your reactivity in your thoughts, emotions, and bodily responses and disengage from it, or witness it.

2. *Refocus* your physiological response by releasing the muscles in your eyes and shoulders, dropping your attention to your torso, and establishing a grounded breathing pattern.

3. *Nurture.* Hold yourself in a state of loving connection to the life that is possible and assure yourself that you deserve all it has to offer. Pay attention to specific details and let yourself *feel* the experience. As vividly as you can, hold this image and experience the loving connection and hope it generates.

The following practice is a variation and uses the HEART protocol to nurture a sense of clarity. It can be used to foster clarity on a specific issue or more general directions for your life.

Variation: HEART for Clarity. HEART for Clarity uses the basic steps of the HEART for Hope protocol above with the intention of gaining clarity on a specific question, problem, or issue.

Before you begin the practice, write down a question, issue, problem, or any life circumstance you would like some clarity on. During the practice, do not overtly focus on this question, just go into the practice with the intention of holding a subconscious awareness of this question. After the practice, notice any answers, intuitive insights, bodily sensations, or other ways of knowing that may surface. These knowings may appear in a variety of ways. Be open. Pay attention. Write down the first things that come up without conscious filtering. Let your writing lead you. In addition, pay attention in the hours and days following the practice. Answers and clarity may emerge at the times you least expect it.

Maintenance. Spend at least ten minutes every day reflecting on what went well and why. Practice HEART for Hope at least once a week and HEART for Clarity when called to do so. Make sure to record your experiences in a practice log.

CONCLUSION: LIVING THE SCIENCE OF HEARTFULNESS

In this chapter, you deepened your engagement with heartful emotion. You read about the powerful benefits of gratitude, empathy, compassion, hope, and the myriad of ways research has shown them to counterbalance stress. You have learned about the impediments to the effective practice of these specific emotions, learned a program to overcome those impediments, and actively participated in their prescriptions in your own life. Specifically, you learned that for gratitude to be beneficial, it must be authentically felt, not coerced or pretended, and you engaged in activities for its genuine practice. You experienced the deep and healing potential of empathy and compassion, both for yourself and for your relationships, by rescripting your emotional past and the difficult emotions "below the line." And, finally, you cultivated hope by seeing yourself beyond the struggle and brought attention to your own personal power to get you there.

The healing benefits of these prescriptive emotions are dependent on how much they are practiced, and you will ever deepen their healing potential by integrating them and practicing them in your daily life. For a new experience to heal, it must be practiced often enough and deep enough to replace the old experience. The more you engage in the activities presented in this chapter, the more efficacy they will produce.

The next section invites you into implementing heartful engagement in the very fabric of your life. It invites you to make it your lived experience through your time, stories, and values. It invites you to be intentional about how you would like your life to "speak."

part 3

Taking It to the Next Level

In part 1, you gained an understanding of stress in general and what your stress response looks and acts like when it is out of control, or on a downward spiral. You were also introduced to the concept of recognizing, releasing, and replacing through mindful awareness and heartful engagement, and to the possibility of what your spiral could look like when it is flowing in an upward direction, or under the influence of your calm-and-connection system. In part 2, you learned the skills of implementation. You learned to recognize and release an out-of-control fear response. You also intentionally activated your calm-and-connection system by replacing your reactivity with heartful engagement and specific prescriptions for heartful emotions to begin the process of deeper restoration. In part 3, you will further this process by restoring your capacities for resilience and well-being, indeed, leading to true flourishing. As such, you will learn and apply what it takes to take it to the next level by integrating and assimilating these concepts in your life as a whole. You will look at what it takes to "let your life speak" and move forward with a transformed self-image.

chapter 6

Restore Your Capacities for Resilience and Flourishing

People are born with innate capacities for emotional resilience and flourishing. *Resilience* is the ability to fully and quickly bounce back from life's emotional difficulties and flourishing is that state of thriving and growing where you are reaching your full potential. Unfortunately, although most people are born with these capacities, they have been largely lost, or never given the chance to grow. Your life's circumstances may have blocked their development in the first place; or, because of your life's stresses, they may have been diminished, or they may have disappeared altogether.

Most of this book has facilitated for you a process to reclaim the foundation for those capacities through reducing your fear-response system and fully establishing the dominance of calm and connection in your life. In this chapter, you will further your process of personal restoration; you will more fully restore your capacities for resilience and flourishing through an intentional implementation of heartful engagement in your everyday life. Further, you will reflect on how this personal restoration might be enacted in your values and the very way you live.

First, you will examine the power and implications of the narratives you tell and the scripts you write and be invited to tell different stories. We all tell "stories," privately and out loud. These stories are based on how you see the world and your position in it. Even after much of the directed healing you experienced throughout the last several chapters have taken hold, some of the stories may remain. They are the more subtle and insidious ways stress prevents you from fully thriving and restoring new life. Unfortunately, these stories are often built on errone-ous concepts of yourself and the world, but have become so ingrained that you are not even aware you are living them. Further, you write "scripts" based on your expectations that only make them more likely to manifest. In other words, you expect certain outcomes from the events or people that are the subjects of your stories and, unintentionally, create those outcomes by your behavior.

You will first explore how you formulate these stories through your interpretation of specific events, both while they are happening and after they have occurred, and delve into alternative, more life-giving versions. Second, you will also look at some of the stories you have for-mulated around who you are and the scripts you write for yourself and then rewrite them with new promise. Finally, you will look at the stories you tell and scripts you write for others. Your expectation of others, often unintentionally, determines your behavior toward them and limits their behavior in response. Simply put, they behave in the way you expect because they are playing the role you have written for them.

After you have assessed the powerful impact of your stories and how you might begin to rewrite a new narrative for your life, you will be invited to look at the power and potential of how you spend your time. The fact that every moment of every day you are transforming to more of the same underscores the importance of how you spend all your moments. Are those moments filled with things that give you life or things that deplete it? You will be invited to examine this question and find ways to fill your moments with more life-generating activities, people, conversations, and so forth as opposed to life-depleting ones. You will identify and implement what, for you, are paths to vitality through mere time and energy commitment.

Next, you will explore how you would most like your life to speak. Through a series of deep reflective exercises, you will consider your life's most meaningful values and explore how they might play out in the way you live your life. You will look at the qualities you most want to embody, the things in your life that are most significant for you in which to dedi-cate your time and energy, and how you want to be remembered.

Finally, from all the exercises in this chapter, you will develop a visual image of the person you most want to be and bring forward into the world. This vision is the basis for the chapter's culminating practice. It is designed to cement, in your body, your mind, and your brain—indeed your whole mind-body complex—a new, embodied, and lived self-image, one that exists beyond the stress and anxiety that may have consumed you and embodies emotional resilience, peace, and well-being.

However, before we move on, it is important to visit the concept of willingness. Without a true willingness to actually *be* different, cultivating emotional resilience and well-being is just a lofty goal. Many times people profess to *want* change, but at a deep level, they are not really willing to make room for it in their life—they are not willing to let go of their old perceptions of themselves and actually embrace a new paradigm.

WILLINGNESS

Unfortunately, with all the self-help knowledge out there, there is an imbalance in the amount of available information and the number of people who actually experience change. In other words, there are many people acquiring knowledge *about* transformation without actually implementing it into their life and reaping the benefits. Change requires action, and action requires willingness. It takes willingness to look at the narratives you tell and the scripts you write about your life events, yourself, and others, and to rewrite those narratives. It takes willingness to look at how you spend your time and to intentionally fill it with more life-generating moments than life-depleting moments. And it takes willingness to look at your deepest held values, or how you would like your life to "speak," and to move forward into the world with a new self-image reflecting those narratives and values. Merely professing to *want* transformation does not work. It takes authentic willingness to truly *be* different and integrate heartful action and maintenance into the very fabric of your life.

As you move forward, it is important to embrace this and acknowledge some of the things that often block people so you can move through those blocks easily. Often, an awareness and acknowledgment of them is all that is needed.

First, from an embodied perspective, change may feel physically unfamiliar—not necessarily bad, just unfamiliar. Because every emotional state carries its corresponding physiological imprint, the new imprints you are embodying carry new physical sensations throughout your body as well. As bad for you and uncomfortable as stressed-out states are, unfortunately, they feel somewhat familiar. The new calm sensation of oxytocin *feels* different from the stressed-out states of cortisol. You need time to adapt to a new baseline state of homeostasis with the new, more healthy, embodied states. All it takes is a little acknowledgment that the physical unfamiliarity is actually a very, very good thing, as is the ability to embrace its newness. Soon you will get used to routinely feeling good!

Second, to adapt to new and restorative stories, you need to be willing to let go of the old. To fully embrace new self-images, in all aspects of your life, you need to be able to let go of the old, possibly ingrained, and subtle perceptions of yourself you may carry in a variety of circumstances. These are the sly stories that you may play out without overt conscious awareness. Intentionally bringing your awareness to them and acknowledging them helps you move beyond them and begin to tell new ones.

Lastly, it is important to examine the payoffs in staying stuck. Most of the time, the benefits of moving forward far, far outweigh the ones of staying stuck, but you may unknowingly self-sabotage your transformative efforts if you are not consciously aware of those of remaining in status quo. In other words, you unintentionally block your success because of some unrealized reward by staying stuck. For example, you may think you don't have opportunities at work, when in reality, what motivates you is the pay-off in staying stuck: you don't have to risk trying. When you bring these subconscious stuck rewards to conscious awareness and realize they are dwarfed by the benefits of moving forward, your self-sabotaging behavior diminishes. You consciously examine the payoffs of staying stuck, make a deliberate choice to move forward, and take appropriate action.

Once you have acknowledged the feeling of physical newness that will accompany you and the need to let go of old stories to make room for the new, have examined them, and have moved beyond the subconscious payoffs of staying stuck, you are ready to take the next steps to personal restoration.

Behavior change theorists break transformation into stages, and although the first few stages involve learning about and planning the desired change, nothing really happens until the action and maintenance stages. Based on the foundations of your willingness, this chapter builds on the actions you started through the skills and practices in part 2 and leads you through a process of integration in your life as a whole. This process of integration will help you restore your capacities for resilience by broadening the actions of your heartful engagement through fresh narratives, time considerations, and a new self-image. It will lead you through a process of incorporating them into your life and maintaining their presence as you move forward to a new and heartful paradigm. This chapter is also deeply experiential, and giving yourself the necessary time and focus to engage in the material is paramount.

CHANGE YOUR STORIES

Personal restoration requires seeing with new eyes or telling new stories. I love the quote "When you change the way you look at things, the things you look at change" (Dyer 2007). That saying fits with what I am referring to here as your "stories." Your stories are your storied interpretations of the current events of your life, your role in them, and the roles of others. As true as they may seem, they are a subjective interpretation based on your "programming," perceptions, and past experience. I am not referring to the past autobiographical events of your life, although you can entertain them here, too, if it is appropriate; what I am referring to is the way you see and interpret your present and the stories you tell around it.

"Things are always like that," "This is just the role I play," "I'm never good enough," "I'm just not meant to succeed in this area," and

"People will always leave me," may represent some of the general interpretations you build your stories around. The problem with many of
your stories is they don't leave room for growth. They may be built from
some true past experience, but through your retelling or reliving them,
they take on a life of their own and perpetuate their presence in your
life. We all subjectively interpret our life and build stories around those
interpretations. They also can be built from the way we interpret the
events themselves.

CHANGE YOUR STORIES AROUND EVENTS

Unfortunately, you may often and unknowingly expect the worst in
events, and those expectations form the outcome. Or, you may look for
any evidence that your skewed interpretations are, in fact, reality, and
proceed accordingly. For some people, it is like they are on high alert for
the worst to happen. How many times have you seen someone take an
event that was 80 to 90 percent positive, obsess on the 10 percent that
they perceived wasn't, and then evaluate the whole event as being
harmful or worthless? The problem in those types of situations is that
the negative evaluation determines future outcomes. Worse, their brain
solidifies and cements the neural networks associated with the negative
interpretation. They are literally training their brain to see more of the
same.

There is hope, however. Most often, you have multiple ways you can
interpret circumstances, and the interpretation itself changes the
outcome. I once had two friends who could walk into the same room
full of people and have completely different experiences. One would
walk in and see all the dysfunction; they could see all the things "wrong"
with the people in the room. The second person could walk in and see
all the gifts of the people in the room. Same room. Same people. Two
completely different interpretations.

The important point here is that both stories were true, but the
person who perceived the room full of gifts had a completely different
and much more generative experience, and she responded in kind. She,

ultimately, formed closer relationships with the people she encountered in that room and created constructive experiences from there. She also, then, was building a stronger foundation to live from that space. Imagine this happening over and over again to where your very perceptions begin to be molded by your routine experience.

Further, your interpretation of the moment activates either your fear-response system or your calm-and-connection system, and which system is in control momentarily can profoundly change the moments that follow. As I describe in the story below, this was once brought home for me in a powerful way because I knew if my fear-response system became dominant, it could be a very dangerous situation for me and my children. Although this is a singular example, these opportunities play out for us every day; it is your *interpretation* of events that can transform them into more memorable experiences. As you read, think of instances in your everyday life, your work, your family life, and your relational life that might lend themselves to changed experiences by your different interpretations of them.

My kids and I used to love to take road trips. Music was always a crucial part of these trips as we would drive down the road and sing at the top of our lungs. The music kept me awake and alert and all of us engaged in a fun and celebratory atmosphere. I would spend hours before every trip just getting the perfect mix of music prepared.

Once, when my kids were still fairly young, we were heading out on a road trip through the desert. I wanted to make sure we left early enough to get through the dangerous part of a two-lane highway before dark. I also wanted to make sure we got far enough to find a place to spend the night because in the desert, there were not many choices. Thankfully, I had many hours of music ready to keep me attentive.

Everything that could go wrong started to go that way, from traffic, to a flat tire, to witnessing an accident on the highway, and I was beginning to worry about our timing. It was already dark, we were just heading into the desert, and we still had many hours to go. We were out in the middle of nowhere, and the music broke. And it started to rain quite heavily. And we had no cell phone reception. Worse, when we got to our planned destination, we found a town with absolutely no vacancies in any motel within many miles.

I knew if I got upset and my brain got flooded with cortisol, I would not be able to think clearly and would become overwhelmed with the situation. I also knew that my kids would become upset, and one of them suffered from high levels of anxiety. It was very important to keep the three of us in a calm and connected state of mind, for we had hours to go and very rough conditions to go through. They were little and scared, and so was their mother.

Trying to figure out how to keep us all calm, I invited them to look at everything that was going wrong in a humorous light. I was also pointing out all the things that we could be grateful for, and we made it a game to find the good, or opportunity, in every challenge. Soon we were actually laughing at all the setbacks, making up fun stories around them, and engaging in a whole different way. We were genuinely having a great time. We decided that since the music was broken, we could sing instead. Unfortunately, the only songs we could remember were Christmas carols, and it was August! So, there we continued, driving down the highway for many more hours, in the dark, in the desert, in the rain, playing our "grateful game," laughing, and singing Christmas carols at the top of our lungs on a memorable August night.

To this day, although it could have been a disastrous situation for all of us, it is still one of our favorite memories.

Much of the time, you have a choice about how to interpret events. Often both interpretations are true; however, the one you focus on is the one that begins to determine your subsequent moments. This is called "subjective interpretation." Subjective interpretation means you are interpreting events through your individual perception. A heartful and embodied approach to subjective interpretation is not about sup-pressing that which needs to be healed; it is about embracing heartful opportunities when authentically possible and appropriate.

Exercise and Reflection: Bring a Heartful Approach to Your Subjective Interpretation

Genuinely and honestly reflect on your tendencies in the area of sub-jective interpretation. What stories do you tell when multiple versions are possible? What specific events or situations in your life could change with a different interpretation? If it feels comfortable to do so, pick a specific event that you could have interpreted differently and reflect how the outcome might have been different. Write in a stream-of-consciousness style, and process and reflect in a way that is appro-priate for you. Additionally, you can be preemptive about the future. What are some future situations that you typically see one way that might lend themselves to a different, more generative interpretation?

Beyond the stories you tell of events, you often tell stories about yourself and others. Further, you write scripts based on your expecta-tions of resultant behavior, and these stories and scripts become self-perpetuating. They are based on your perceptions and are also subjective, although not always obviously so. You may want to believe that you or someone else just *are* a certain way, but being open to changing the story or allowing another narrative to develop is the first step to growth.

CHANGE YOUR STORIES ABOUT YOURSELF AND OTHERS

You are constantly constructing your reality with your words, thoughts, and stories. You tell stories about yourself, you tell stories about others, and you tell stories about your relationships. Sometimes they are verbal, but most often, they are held as your own internal narrative, and this narrative has power. You begin to believe them, fortify them, and per-petuate them.

Further, even when there is some truth to a story, there are usually multiple stories surrounding it. The story you tell might only be a partial piece, but it is made the only story by the way you tell it. If both are true and the one you tell becomes your reality, you may want to rethink your narratives. They may not even be "true." Or, they may have some truth, but not be completely true. Or, they may be true now, but the longer you continue to tell them, the less room you give to grow beyond them. Also, because your fear-response system is often dominant, if you are not aware, the threat-based story will be the story that is more prominent.

Your stories form and perpetuate who you are and who others in your life are, and you tell your stories from a selective truth. You are in a constant feedback loop with the stories you tell and the scripts you write, and the only way to restore new life is to be open to and tell new stories.

Sometimes, when I am in conversation with my husband, I realize I am telling a narrative of who I expect him to be in that moment. It may be based on some past truth or my skewed perceptions, but it leaves no room for him to be anything different. In reality, I am creating the outcome by my expectations. The truth is, I have multiple narratives of who he may be at any given moment, and they are most often based on my own momentary perceptions and embodied state. When I can tell the story of who he is at his core and expect that person to show up, he most often does.

Beyond your stories, you have scripts of your expected outcomes. These are the ways you play out your narratives, write the outcome, and perpetuate the expected reality. Your scripts, just like your stories, may be based on a false or skewed interpretation of reality, yet you play them out as if they were absolutely true. You are giving yourself, or others, a certain role to play, complete with scripted behavior. When you write scripts for others, you often unknowingly manifest what you expect. In other words, you anticipate and then act as if what you expect is a given outcome.

Regina was a very bright and capable young woman. She seemingly had everything going for her but was absolutely convinced that every time she walked into a room, everybody was judging her. This was an issue in her work because she often made public presentations.

Although she should have been well on her way to professional success, the anxiety around feeling judged was crippling her; she told herself this story so many times that she did not leave open the possibility for another outcome. The ironic thing is that people generally loved her presentations, except they noticed that she seemed nervous about being judged.

Exercise and Reflection: Rewrite Your Stories and Scripts

What are the narratives or stories you tell about yourself? About others? What are the scripts that you write for yourself or others? What would happen if you let go of some of your limiting stories? Are you allowing room for growth or another, more heartful story to be told? Write in a stream-of-consciousness style addressing some of the above questions. Remember the more you deeply engage, the more room you provide for transformation.

Opportunities to change your stories and write new scripts play themselves out every day in the tapestry of your life. Every day you are provided with new openings, tangible and specific ways to live a new narrative. What if you could write new stories and scripts for the way you interpret your life and life's events?

Sandy, a workshop participant, told a funny story about a moment of awakening for her. She had been struggling with many life issues, yet they were limited and defined by the stories of who she thought she was. She was in the shower one day and had an absolute moment of aha! After processing about her own stories and scripts in our workshop, it hit her like a ton of bricks that she simply did not have to keep telling those stories. She realized she was completely free to start telling new ones. All it took was a little acknowledgment because, in the end, they were just her stories.

Letting go of old stories leaves space to create fresh ones. The process of personal restoration through heartful engagement invites you now to reflect on how you might spend your time with renewed stories.

EXAMINE YOUR TIME BUDGET AND ENERGY DEPOSITS

You only have so much time in a day. Further, every moment of time is a moment of experience. Recall that, as a "system of adaptation," you are transforming to every moment's experience, whether you are aware or not. So, the more your moments are filled with life-degenerating activities, or even status quo activities, the more your stress response remains the same; the more your moments are filled with life-generating activities, the more you rewire to a life of vitality and well-being. Imagine you have a "time budget" and you need to decide how to best spend your valuable time.

Looking at time this way places a whole new level of personal responsibility on what you do with the moments of your life. If all the moments of your time are valuable and ultimately transforming (good or bad), how do you spend them? What do the moments of your days consist of? Transformation is not only designated to those moments when you feel like it or are on retreat, vacation, or a specifically targeted path; it is the result of the accumulation of all the moments of your life. And when you keep in mind that every moment carries a physiological imprint that delivers the capacity for more of the same, you realize the cumulative power of how you spend *all* those moments.

In this section, you will be invited to identify your energy-draining moments and your energy-enhancing moments. From an embodied perspective, those moments that are energy-draining carry the physiological imprint of life degeneration, and those moments that are energy-enhancing carry the physiological imprint of life generation. Simply put, they impact the direction of your spiral of becoming accordingly. In the next exercise, you will consider the impact of these moments in terms of the people, places, and events that occupy them. It is important to note, however, that there are no universal answers. What may be energy draining for you may not necessarily be the same for another. It is also important to note that looking at time this way does not demand you to be perfect all the time. It is about balance, awareness, and tipping the scales, more often than not, to life-generating activities.

Exercise and Reflection: Shift Your Time and Energy to Life Generation

Following are some common considerations that may add to or detract from your personal energy stores. This is, in no way, meant to be an exhaustive list. It is meant to help you explore how this phenomenon plays out in your own life. Consider the following, but also consider what may be personal "energy influencers" in your own life. Remember, the type of energy you expose yourself to determines the embodied experience of the moment, and the embodied experience of all your moments becomes your life.

How do the people in your life contribute to or detract from your personal energy stores? Admittedly, there are those that you have no choice about, but there are others you do. Think about the relationships in your life: the more pronounced ones and the ones you have lesser contact with. How do you feel when you are engaged in these relationships? What is your authentic embodied response when you are in their presence? Take a few moments and reflect. Close your eyes, rest in the physical sensations of your body, and imagine the various people in your life. Notice how your physical sensations shift when different people are brought into your awareness. Be sure to stay with the sensations long enough so you know your embodied response is a genuine one, not just an immediate reaction. How can you maximize your time and contact with the people who nurture a sense of generation and lessen contact with those who do not? If you cannot change your exposure to some people in your life who are energy draining, how can you shift your interaction with them to reduce their impact?

What about media? Which forms of media leave you with a feeling of life-generation, and which do not? Are you a person who is particularly sensitive to the media exposure in your life? Think about media in all forms in your life and remember that your brain does not know the difference between what is vividly imagined and what is real. Think about the various movie, television, computer, and smartphone interactions you have each day or just the amount of time you spend involved with them, and reflect on how they make you feel from a deeply embodied perspective. What shifts are you called to make?

Reflect on your environment and how sensitive you are to the space that surrounds you. Environmental concerns can include everything from your immediate environment to the time you spend in nature. What is your embodied reaction when you think of your environmental needs? What are your needs for simplicity? Do you need more simplicity in your environment? Do you need more simplicity in life in general? Many of the moments that you spend overly stimulated by your environment, your countless demands, and your latest acquisitions might be better spent in more life-generating activities and places. Could you benefit from voluntary simplicity in which you make a conscious choice to reduce the inner and outer clutter in your life?

How can you be more intentional about self-care and personal time? Remember that your time budget is made up of the moments of your life, and the more you spend your moments on life-generating activities, the more you transform. How can you extend this concept to the personal care of your physical body, as in nutrition and exercise? Reflect on ways you might allocate more time to the things that feed you on a deeper level. Do you have enough silence or contemplative practice in your life? Do you make sure you dedicate time to generative or inspired activities, and what do those look like for you? Do you spend time processing and exploring the synchronicities that show up in your life? Are you taking time to foster meaningful connections? To laugh? To smile? All these things create the biochemical shifts throughout your body and brain that engage your calm-and-connection system and rewire your stress response at a fundamental level. How can you incorporate more of them in your life?

Think about your time as a valuable commodity and an investment in who you are becoming. After reflecting on what you just read, identify what shifts can you make to allocate more time to those things that are, for you, life-generating. What specific steps can you take to incorporate them into more moments of your life? Write in a stream-of-consciousness style, and process and reflect in a way that is appropriate for you.

Renovating what you spend your time and energy on creates a calmer baseline of homeostasis and opens up spaces for deeper transformation. Once you have genuinely reflected on the value of every present moment, you will now look at the "you" that you would most like to bring forward into those moments, or how you would most like your life "to speak."

DISCOVER AND LIVE YOUR DEEPEST VALUES

Throughout this book, you have seen that reducing your fear-response system and developing your calm-and-connection system leads to a sense of expansiveness in the way that you see and live your life. As you do so, you become more capable of living a life consistent with your deeper values and embodying those values in your everyday life. Letting your life speak by the way you live your deepest held values increasingly expands and solidifies your spiral of becoming; the more integrated and embodied those values are, the more your mind-body complex adapts and responds with an ever-increasing life-generative cycle. Your orb of heartful engagement expands and develops the capacity to absorb more of your life and the lives of those around you. The next section's exercises invite you into a heartful and meaningful look at what those values are for you, clarifying for you how you would most like your life to speak.

They are very loosely based on a combination of activities developed by Stephen Covey (Covey 2013) and Alan Lakein (Lakein 1989).

> *Imagine this: You walk into a space that is immediately impactful. It might be a building, a sanctuary, or somewhere outside; wherever it is, it is a space that represents the deepest parts of who you are. You are not quite sure what type of event you are being invited to attend. You pause, look around, and take it all in. You are confused, a little apprehensive, but mostly very intrigued, as the energy of the space feels like home and connected to the deepest sense of who you are.*
>
> *As you look around, you more fully focus on the various people in attendance. They are from all walks of your life. They somehow represent different aspects of your life that comprise who you are. They represent facets of how you have known them and how you have lived your life—your closest loved ones, extended family, vocational involvements, brief acquaintances, and so forth. You focus on this for a moment and let it sink in. As the significance of the space sinks in, you realize it is completely representative of you and your life. Almost instantaneously, you see some sort of an altar on which there are pictures of you, and you realize that it is a celebration of your life because you have passed on from it! You have walked into your own memorial service.*
>
> *This causes you to deeply pause and ponder a moment as you see people from these various walks of your life preparing to give eulogies. What will they say? What would you want them to say?*

The next exercise is divided into two parts. The different parts are designed to be to done together and in sequence. They will help you better clarify your deepest held values and build your life accordingly.

Part 1: Write Your Eulogy

Take a few deep breaths and imagine yourself in the above scenario. Pick three or four dimensions of your life and write a brief eulogy from the point of view of the person that best represents that dimension. In other words, you are writing from the point of view of someone who may be a close family member, a colleague, or someone who has had a significant impact in another dimension of your life. You are writing the eulogy for yourself. It is based on what you would *like* them to be able to say in celebration of your life. What would you like these various people to be able to say about you, who you were, and how you lived your life? At the end of the eulogy, include fifteen descriptive words or short phrases that you would *like* people to be able to use to describe you and how you lived your life. After you have listed fifteen, reflect on what you wrote, and circle the five that are most meaningful for you.

The above exercise is designed to help you gain clarity on your deepest values and what is truly important for you to embody in this life. However, even when you are aware of your deepest values, you may not be embodying them in your day-to-day experience as well as you might be. You might be, as people often are, waiting until "things calm down," you finish this endeavor or that project, or you get done with a specific phase of your life (school, relationship, job, into retirement) to truly live your values. Unfortunately, I know people well into their very advanced years that are still waiting for their life to begin. A life of heartful engagement invites you in to a life based on your deepest values—right now. Imagine the following:

An angel has just visited you. Her message for you is that your time is finite. She has come to let you know that you only have a year left to live. You will not be sick, and you do not have to spend the year getting your affairs in order. Her message is not meant to be morbid in any way. In fact, it is the greatest gift she can give you (other than longer life). It is meant to be the gift of knowing that your time is short so in that knowing, you can spend the year in the most meaningful ways to you that are possible. How would you spend that precious time? What would you do with the days and the moments that you have left?

Part 2: How Would You Spend a Year Left to Live? What Did You Learn?

From a place of heartful awareness, imagine you only have a year left to live. You are well, but know your time is finite and short. You want to live that year from your deepest values and have it reflect all that you want to be and do in that time. What would you do? How would you spend that year? Again, write in a stream-of-consciousness style in a way that is appropriate for you.

After you are done with the eulogies, including the descriptive phrases, and writing on your remaining year, reflect on what you wrote. What did you learn about what you most value? How will you incorporate these values into your life? Be specific. Process and reflect in a way that is appropriate for you, understanding that the more detailed you can be about the way you will implement them in a tangible way in your life, the more likely you will be successful at doing so.

Solidifying your new self-image—the one you have identified through examining the importance of where you spend your time and energy; the new stories you are willing to tell about events, yourself, and others; and how you would most like your life to speak—is the next step in rewiring a new way of living.

This last HEART practice invites you into moving forward with a new self-image. It is built from and contains the components of memory reconsolidation as outlined in the previous chapter, but this time, you will be working with a more generalized self-image. This self-image will reflect and solidify what you learned in this chapter and foster a new sense of resilience and flourishing as you move forward in your life. Reflect on the activities within this chapter; it might be helpful to reread some of your reflections. Ponder deeply about what you would look like if you were truly embodying what you wrote. What would your life look like if you were truly spending your time in life-generating ways? What would your new stories and narratives convey? How would you realize and live your identified values?

Practice: HEART for a New You

To listen to a recording of this practice, go to http://www.newharbinger.com/42839. Take some time before the practice and get extremely clear on an image or components of different images you would like to bring forth and the way you would like your life to speak. Briefly reflect on the images you want to leave behind, just enough to unlock the associated neural networks and destabilize them. Again, and importantly, it is enough to just bring them to mind without letting them consume you or your emotional equilibrium. Next, bring to mind your new and desired self-image and engage in the following.

1. *Notice* your reactivity in your thoughts, emotions, and bodily responses and disengage from it, or witness it.

2. *Refocus* your physiological response by releasing the muscles in your eyes and shoulders, dropping your attention to your torso, and establishing a grounded breathing pattern.

3. *Nurture:* Hold a picture of yourself truly embodying your new self-image. Imagine yourself in the details of this perception, as this will solidify the encoding of the new image. Notice the sounds, smells, and sights, and especially focus on the *felt experience* of the new image. It is okay if it is not static, if it moves and shifts. You may have pieces of the image shift and come in and out of conscious awareness; that is fine; most images actually are dynamic. The important thing is that you rest in the felt experience and notice the details when they do come up. As deeply and as honestly as you can, fully immerse yourself in the vision and sensation of this new image. Hold it as long as it is comfortable, or for fifteen to twenty minutes.

After the practice, if you are called to do so, journal about your experience. This can solidify the practice even more. It is also important to come out of the practice slowly and reflect as you do because doing so integrates the more conscious parts of your brain with the parts that just experienced the practice. Journaling helps you recall the experience of the practice in the more conscious moments of your day and act accordingly. Soak in the richness of the experience.

The more you engage in any practice, the more it rewires you to a new way of resilience and well-being. The more you engage in this practice, the more fully you will embody your new self-image and bring it forth into your new life.

CONCLUSION: FROM INTENT TO ACTION

This chapter has been deeply experiential, and it is important to spend some time soaking in the experience of the last practice. It is also important that you revisit it and the material in this chapter often; doing so will more fully embody its content in the intentionality of your life.

You looked at the stories you tell about events, yourself, and others and were invited to tell new ones, ones that would better contribute to the life you want to bring forth from here. Through your considerations of time and energy, you realized at a tangible level that the things that most occupy your moments are the things that become the foundation of your life. You were invited to look at what these things are and at their energy potential—whether they contribute to life generation or life depletion for you. You also examined your deepest values—the ones you would most want people to remember you by and the ones you would live if your time were finite.

Finally, you deeply experienced a new self-image based on all the considerations in this chapter and book and encoded that image in your body and mind. With this new self-image, you can more effectively move in to a life of personal restoration; one full of resilience and flourishing.

Conclusion: Moving Forward

As you come to the end of this book, my hope is that your process is just beginning. All the content, skills, writings, and deeper practices in this book were designed to bring you from a fear-dominated, downward spiral in your emotional life to an upward spiral of calm and connection, leading you to heightened states of resilience and well-being. However, the journey is just beginning. And ultimately, it never ends.

Behavior change is often broken down into steps, and at its heart are the steps of contemplation, action, maintenance, and "accidentally quitting." Although there is not always a completely defined border between the steps, the *contemplation* stage includes understanding the problem and laying the foundation for change—in essence, preparing for transformation. Part 1 of this book offered you that.

The next stage is *action*, and nothing really transforms until this stage takes place. Again, one of my favorite sayings is "Nothing changes, if nothing changes." The rest of the book invited you into action and change. Through the skills, writings, and practices, you engaged in a different paradigm for your emotional life, a different experiential way of being. Also, you engaged in a flip of the typical understanding of the cause-and-effect relationship of stress and your emotional life. As a reminder, stress in your external life is often looked at as the cause and the nature of your emotional life, the effect. In reality, it is the other way around. In this book, you have worked to change your external life by changing your internal life through the profound impact of heartful emotion and all its implications for transformation.

Now is the *maintenance* phase. This phase is as important as the original action phase because now, you find a way to make heartful engagement a part of your everyday existence and weave it into the fabric of your life. The journaling and HEART practices in this book were not designed to be done only once or twice; the more you make them a part of your daily life, the more transformative they will ulti-mately be. It is your job now to find a way to integrate them in your life to keep reaping their benefits. Be creative, honor what works for you, but do continue.

Also, it is important to have some understanding of the next phase: accidentally quitting. Accidentally quitting is exactly as it sounds. For some reason or another, life often presents a challenge: sickness, work demand, or other event that gets in the way of your everyday practice. A day becomes a week, a week becomes two, and you realize you have quit without intending to. Just understanding that this concept is "a thing," and planning ahead for it, often relieves it. True behavior and foundational life change is far more about getting back on the horse than being perfect in the first place. It is about continually restoring the action and maintenance phases and always bringing yourself back to the truth and transformational power of heartful emotion and the skills and practices to get you there.

Lastly, and most importantly, a word about love. In this book, you learned and experienced the life-changing powers of intentionally engaging in heartful emotion overall and the specific transformative power of gratitude, empathy, compassion, and hope. Love is the state that encompasses it all.

Although love often precludes a specific definition—the deeper something is felt, the fewer words there are that can describe it—it is the state that encompasses, deepens, and continually widens the prac-tice of all the heartful emotions. As stated in the introduction, its purpose is to ever grow and extend outward all the inner transforma-tions you have experienced through this process. Heartful engagement is an ever-deepening process for you, but also an ever-widening opportu-nity to encompass it all in love and extend that love outward.

It has been my deep, deep honor to be the facilitator of this process for you, and my wish for you is that now you make it your own, deeply weave it into the fabric of your life, and send it out in ever-widening circles. Like a pebble dropped in a still pond, may your experience with heartful emotion continually transform you and the love that results embrace ever-expanding spheres.

In love,

Alane

Acknowledgments

I am grateful for so many different people that played a part in helping me see this book to fruition. The strength in most things in life is the interdependence and connections that help create them. My gratitude spans from people who helped with the specifics of the book's creation, to those who have engaged in the journey of its content, to those who play an ever-supportive role in my life.

First, to the folks at New Harbinger. Thank you for believing in the idea initially and in helping form and reform its contents along the way. Thank you, also, to the many, many students and workshop and retreat attendees who have shared your journey with me. I am truly blessed to do what I do and be invited to witness such a sacred process of self-transformation. I can't express enough how much the sharing in your processes has meant to me. I am grateful too, to the Cal Poly College of Science and my Love Button family. My heart is full in appreciation for your support. Thank you, too, to those who have played a role in keeping me balanced and lending endless encouragement, both in lessening the workload of the lab so I had time to write and playing the part of cheerleader for my work. To all my lab assistants, thank you. And an especially heartfelt thank-you to Justin Gaytan.

Thank you, too, to my family. The memories of both my parents ever sustain me with their support. Thank you to my siblings, who are not only my siblings, but my best friends; my stepson Justin; and my sons Michael and Sammy, always an integral part of who I am.

Finally, to my husband Frank. Thank you for your support, encouragement, love, sustaining belief in me, time in Hana, and all the immeasurable ways we have grown together. I love you.

References

Agren, T. 2014. "Human Reconsolidation: A Reactivation and Update." *Brain Research Bulletin* 105. https://doi.org/10.1016/j.brainresbull.2013.12.010.

Algoe, S. B., B. L. Fredrickson, and S. L. Gable. 2013. "The Social Functions of the Emotion of Gratitude via Expression." *Emotion* 4 (August 2013): 605–609.

Algoe, S. B., and B. M. Way. 2014. "Evidence for a Role of the Oxytocin System, Indexed by Genetic Variation in CD38, in the Social Bonding Effects of Expressed Gratitude." *Social, Cognitive and Affective Neuroscience* 9 (12): 1855–1861. https://doi.org/10.1093/scan/nst182.

Arntz, A. 2012. "Imagery Rescripting as a Therapeutic Technique: Review of Clinical Trials, Basic Studies, and Research Agenda." *Journal of Experimental Psychopathology* 3 (2): 189–208. https://doi.org/10.5127/jep.024211.

Ashar, Y. K., J. R. Andrews-Hanna, S. Dimidjian, and T. D. Wager. 2016. "Towards a Neuroscience of Compassion: A Brain Systems-Based Model and Research Agenda." In *Positive Neuroscience*, edited by J. D. Greene, I. Morrison, and M. E. Seligman, 125–141. New York: Oxford University Press.

Ashby, F. G., A. M. Isen, and A. U. Turken. 1999. "Neurophysiological Theory of Positive Affect and Its Influence on Cognition." *Psychological Review* 106 (3): 529–550.

Balkie, K. A., and K. Wilhelm. 2005. "Emotional and Physical Health Benefits of Expressive Writing." *Advances in Psychiatric Treatment* 11: 338–346.

Begley, S. 2007. *Train Your Mind, Change Your Brain: How a New Science Reveals Our Extraordinary Potential to Transform Ourselves.* New York: Ballantine Books.

Bos, P. A., E. R. Montoya, E. J. Hermans, C. Keysers, and J. Van Honk. 2015. "Oxytocin Reduces Neural Activity in the Pain Circuitry When Seeing Pain in Others." *Neuroimage* 113 (June): 217–224.

Chen, L. H., M. Y. Chen, and Y. M. Tsai. 2012. "Does Gratitude Always Work? Ambivalence Over Emotional Expression Inhibits the Beneficial Effect of Gratitude on Well-Being." *International Journal of Psychology* (Jan 17): 382–392.

Chrousos, G. P., D. L. Loriaux, and P. W. Gold. 1988. *Mechanisms of Physical and Emotional Stress.* New York: Plenum Press.

Cichy, R. M., J. Heinzle, and J. D. Haynes. 2012. "Imagery and Perception Share Cortical Representations of Content and Location." *Cerebral Cortex* 22 (2): 372–380.

Covey, S. 2013. *The Seven Habits of Highly Effective People (Anniversary Edition).* New York: Simon and Schuster.

Cozolino, L. 2010. *The Neuroscience of Psychotherapy: Healing the Social Brain.* New York: W. W. Norton and Company.

Doane, L. D., and E. K. Adam. 2010. "Loneliness and Cortisol: Momentary, Day-to-Day, and Trait Associations." *Psychoneuroendricrinology* 35 (3): 430–441.

Dyer, W. 2007. *Change Your Thoughts, Change Your Life: Living the Wisdom of the Tao.* Carlsbad, CA: Hay House.

Ecker, B. 2015. "Memory Reconsolidation Understood and Misunderstood." *Internaional Journal of Neuropsychotherapy* 3 (1): 2–46. https://doi.org/10.12744/ijnpt.2015.0002-0046.

Emmons, R. A., and C. A. Crumpler. 2000. "Gratitude as a Human Strength: Appraising the Evidence." *Journal of Social and Clinical Psychology* 19: 56–69.

Emmons, R. A., and M. E. McCullough. (Eds.). 2004. *The Psychology of Gratitude.* New York: Oxford University Press.

Emmons, R. A., and R. Stern. 2013. "Gratitude as a Psychotherapeutic Intervention." *Journal of Clinical Psychology* 69 (8): 846–855.

Fox, G., J. Kaplan, H. Damasio, and A. Damasio. 2015. "Neural Correlates of Gratitude." *Frontiers in Psychology* (September 30).

Fredrickson, B. L. 2013a. *Love 2.0: How Our Supreme Emotion Affects Everything We Feel, Think, Do, and Become.* New York: Hudson Street Press.

Fredrickson, B. L. 2013b. "Positive Emotions Broaden and Build." *Advances in Experimental Social Psychology* 47: 1–53.

Fredrickson, B. L., M. A. Cohn, K. A. Coffey, J. Pek, and S. M. Finkel. 2008. "Open Hearts Build Lives: Positive Emotions, Induced Through Loving Kindness Meditation, Build Consequential Personal Resources." *Journal of Personality and Social Psychology* 95 (5): 1045–1062. https://doi.org/10.1037/a0013262.

Fredrickson, B. L., and R. W. Levinson. 1998. "Positive Emotions Speed Recovery from the Cardiovascular Sequelae of Negative Emotions." *Cognition and Emotion* 12 (2): 191–220.

Fredrickson, B. L., R. A. Mancuso, C. Branigan, and M. M. Tugade. 2000. "The Undoing Effect of Positive Emotions." *Motivation and Emotion* 24 (4): 237–258.

Gendlin, E. 1981. *Focusing.* New York: Bantam Books.

Greenberg, M. S., and D. R. Westcott. 1983. "Indebtedness as a Mediator of Reactions to Aid." In *New Directions in Helping: Recipient Reactions to Aid,* edited by J. Fisher, A. Nadler, and B. M. DePaulo, 85–112. New York: Academic Press.

Guyre, P. M., and A. Munck. 1998. "Glucocorticoids." In *Encyclopedia of Immunology*, edited by P. Delves and I. Roitt, 996–1000. Cambridge, MA: Academic Press.

Harbaugh, C. N., and M. Vasey. 2014. "When Do People Benefit from Gratitude Practice?" *The Journal of Positive Psychology* (June 23): 535–546.

Hillyard, S. A., and L. Anllo-Vento. 1998. "Event-Related Brain Potentials in the Study of Visual Selective Attention." *Proceedings of the National Academy of Sciences of the United States of America*, 95(3): 781–787.

Hofmann, S. G., P. Grossman, and D. E. Hinton. 2011. "Loving Kindness and Compassion Meditation: Potential for Psychological Interventions." *Clinical Psychology Review* 31 (7): 1126–1132. https://doi.org/10.1016/j.cpr.2011.07.003.

Hubbard, J. R., and E. A. Workman, ed. 1998. *The Handbook of Stress: An Organ System Approach*. New York: CRC Press.

Huen, J. M. Y., B. Y. T. Ip, S. M. Ho, and P. S. F. Yip. 2015. "Hope and Hopelessness: The Role of Hope in Buffering the Impact of Hopelessness on Suicidal Ideation." *Public Library of Science* 10 (6).

Isen, A. M., K. A. Daubman, and G. P. Norwicki. 1987. "Positive Affect Facilitates Creative Problem Solving." *Journal of Personal and Social Psychology* 52 (6): 1122–1131.

Kahn, B. E., and A. M. Isen. 1993. "The Influence of Positive Affect on Variety Seeking Among Safe, Enjoyable Products." *Journal on Consumer Research* 20 (2): 257–270.

Kim, J. W., S. E. Kim, J. J. Kim, B. Jeong, C. H. Park, A. R. Son, J. E. Song, and S. W. Ki. 2009. "Compassionate Attitude Towards Others' Suffering Activates the Mesolimbic Neural System." *Neuropsychologia* 47 (10): 2073–2081. https://doi.org/10.1016/j.neuropsychologia.2009.03.017.

Kim, K. J., Y. K. Na, and H. S. Hong. 2016. "Effects of Progressive Muscle Relaxation Therapy in Colorectal Cancer." *Western Journal of Nursing Research* 38 (8): 959–973.

Kirsch, P., C. Esslinger, Q. Chen, D. Mier, S. Lis, S. Siddhanti, H. Gruppe, V. S. Mattay, B. Gallhofer, and A. Meyer-Lindenberg. 2005. "Oxytocin Modulates Neural Circuitry for Social Cognition and Fear in Humans." *Journal of Neuroscience* 25: 11489–11493.

Klimecki, O. M., S. Leiberg, C. Lamm, and T. Singer. 2013. "Functional Neural Plasticity and Associated Changes in Positive Affect after Compassion Training." *Cerebal Cortex* 23 (7): 1552–1561.https://doi .org/10.1093/cercor/bhs142.

Klimecki, O. M., S. Leiberg, S. Ricard, and T. Singer. 2014. "Differential Pattern of Functional Brain Plasticity after Compassion and Empathy Training." *Social, Cognitive and Affective Neuroscience* 9 (6): 873–879. https://doi.org/10.1093/scan/nst060.

Lakein, A. 1989. *How to Get Control of Your Time and Your Life.* New York: Signet Classics.

LeDoux, J. 1993. "Emotional Memory Systems in the Brain." *Behavioral Brain Research* 58 (1-2): 69–79.

LeDoux, J. 2002. *Synaptic Self: How Our Brains Become Who We Are.* New York: Viking Penguin.

LeDoux, J. 2003. "The Emotional Brain, Fear, and the Amygdala." *Cellular and Molecular Neurobiology* 23 (4–5): 727–738.

Leiberg, S., and S. Anders. 2006. "The Multiple Facets of Empathy: A Survey of Theory and Evidence." *Progress in Brain Research* 156: 419–440. https://doi.org/10.1016/S0079-6123(06)56023-6.

Levine, P. 2010. *In an Unspoken Voice: How the Body Releases Trauma and Restores Goodness.* Berkeley: North Atlantic Books.

Losier, M. 2007. *The Law of Attraction: The Science of Attracting More of What You Want, and Less of What You Don't.* New York: Wellness Central.

MacBeth, A., and A. Gumley. 2012. "Exploring Compassion: A Meta-Analysis of the Association Between Self-Compassion and Psychopathology." *Clinical Psychological Review* 32 (6): 545–552.

McCraty, R. 2015. *Science of the Heart, Volume 2.* Boulder Creek, CA: HeartMath, LLC.

McCraty, R., M. Atkinson, W. A. Tiller, G. Rein, and A. D. Watkins. 1995. "The Effect of Emotions on Short-Term Heart Rate Variability Using Power Spectrum Analysis." *American Journal of Cardiology* 76 (14): 1089–1093.

McCraty, R., B. Barrios-Chopin, D. Rozman, M. Atkinson, and A. D. Watkins. 1998. "The Impact of a New Self-Management Program on Stress, Emotions, Heart Rate Variability, DHEA and Cortisol." *Intergated Physiological and Behavioral Science* 33 (2): 151–170.

McNaughton, N. 1989. *Biology and Emotion.* Cambridge: Cambridge University Press.

Neff, K. D., and C. Germer. 2017. "Self-Compassion and Psychological Well-Being." In *Oxford Handbook of Compassion Science*, edited by E. M. Seppälä, E. Simon-Thomas, S. L. Brown, M. C. Worline, C. D. Cameron, and J. R. Doty, 371–386. Oxford: Oxford University Press.

Neisser, U., and I. E. Hyman, Jr. 1982. *Memory Observed.* New York: Worth Publishers.

Ogden, P., K. Minton, and C. Pain. 2006. *Trauma and the Body: A Sensorimotor Approach to Psychotherapy, Interpersonal Neurobiology.* New York: W. W. Norton and Company.

Pennebaker, J. W. 2018. "Expressive Writing in Psychological Writing." *Perspectives on Psychological Science* 13 (2): 226–229.

Peters, M. L., I. K. Flink, K. Boersma, and S. J. Linton. 2010. "Manipulating Optimism: Can Imagining a Best Possible Self Be Used to Increase Future Expectancies?" *Journal of Positive Psychology* 5 (3): 204–211.

Rogers, F., Jr. 2015. *Practicing Compassion*. Nashville: Upper Room Books.

Ruby, P., and J. Decety. 2004. "How Would You Feel Versus How Do You Think She Would Feel? A Neuroimaging Study of Perspective Taking with Social Emotions." *Journal of Cognitive Neuroscience* 19: 988–999.

Sadeghi, H. 2017. *The Clarity Cleanse: 12 Steps to Finding Renewed Energy, Spiritual Fulfillment, and Emotional Healing*. New York: Grand Central Life and Style.

Selye, H. 1936. "A Syndrome Produced by Diverse Nocuous Agents." *Nature* 138 (32): 3479.

Schwartz, R. C. 1997. *Internal Family Systems Therapy*. New York: The Guilford Press.

Seligman, M. E. P. 2011. *Flourish: A Visionary New Understanding of Happiness and Well-Being*. New York: Atria.

Senge, P., J. Schwarmer, and B. S. Flowers. 2004. *Presence: An Exploration of Profound Change in People, Organizations, and Society*. New York: Doubleday.

Siegel, D. J. 2009. "Emotion as Integration." In *The Healing Power of Emotion: Affective Neuroscience, Development and Clinical Practice*, edited by D. Fosha, D. Siegel, and M. Solomon, 145–171. New York: W. W. Norton and Company.

Siegel, D. J. 2010. *Mindsight: The New Science of Personal Transformation*. New York: Bantam Books.

Siegel, D. 2012. *Pocket Guide to Interpersonal Biology: An Integrative Handbook of the Mind*. New York: W. W. Norton & Company.

Singer, T., and O. M. Kilmecki. 2014. "Empathy and Compassion." *Current Biology* 24 (18): R875–R878. https://doi.org/10.1016/j.cub.2014.06.054.

Snyder, C. R. 1989. "Reality Negotiation: From Excuses to Hope and Beyond." *Journal of Clinical and Social Psychology* 8 (2): 130–157.

Van der Kolk, B. A. 2014. *The Body Keeps the Score: Brain, Mind and Body in the Healing of Trauma*. New York: Viking Books.

Van der Kolk, B. A., O. Van der Hart, and C. R. Miramar. 1996. "Disassociation and Information Processing in Post Traumatic Stress Disorder." In *Traumatic Stress: The Effects of Overwhelming Experience on Mind, Body, and Society*, edited by B. A. van der Kolk, A. C. McFarlane, and L. Weisaeth, 303–327. New York: The Guilford Press.

Wood, A. M., J. J. Froh, and A. W. Geraghty. 2010. "Gratitude and Well-Being: A Review and Theoretical Integration." *Clinical Psychology Review* 30 (7). https://doi.org10.1016/j.cpr.2010.03.005.

Wood, A. M., J. Maltby, R. Gillet, P. A. Linley, and S. Joseph. 2008. "The Role of Gratitude in the Development of Social Support, Stress, and Depression: Two Longitudinal Studies." *Journal of Research and Personality* 42 (4): 854–871.

Zak, P. J., R. Kurzban, and W. T. Matzner. 2005. "Oxytocin Is Associated with Human Trustworthiness." *Hormonal Behavior* 48 (5): 522–527.

Zeng, X., C. P. K. Chiu, R.Wang, T. P. S. Oeiu, and F. Y. K. Leung. 2015. "The Effect of Loving-Kindness Meditation on Positive Emotions: A Meta-Analytic Review." *Frontiers in Psychology* 6: 1693.

Alane K. Daugherty, PhD, is a stress expert who teaches courses in stress management, emotional health, embodied spirituality, health and well-being, and the psychophysiology of contemplative practice. She is codirector of the Mind and Heart Research Lab—a psychophysiology lab and stress management and emotional health facility at California Polytechnic State University, Pomona. She also serves as research consultant for the Center for Engaged Compassion at Claremont School of Theology. She routinely speaks and conducts seminars, workshops, and retreats on stress management and cultivating emotional resilience.

Foreword writer **Habib Sadeghi, DO**, is founder of Be Hive of Healing Integrative Medical Center in Agoura Hills, CA. With a master's degree in spiritual psychology, he specializes in treating chronic diseases and their trauma-based, emotional cofactors. He specializes in osteopathic, anthroposophical, environmental, psychosomatic, family, and German new medicine; and integrative psychosynthesis. He is author of *The Clarity Cleanse* and *Within*.

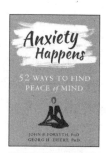
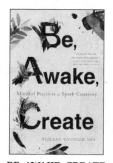
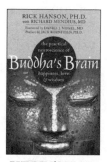
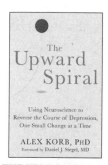
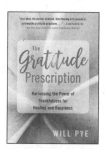
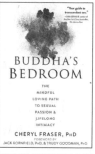
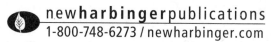

Register your **new harbinger** titles for additional benefits!

When you register your **new harbinger** title—purchased in any format, from any source—you get access to benefits like the following:

- Downloadable accessories like printable worksheets and extra content
- Instructional videos and audio files
- Information about updates, corrections, and new editions

Not every title has accessories, but we're adding new material all the time.

Access free accessories in 3 easy steps:

1. Sign in at NewHarbinger.com (or **register** to create an account).

2. Click on **register a book**. Search for your title and click the **register** button when it appears.

3. Click on the **book cover or title** to go to its details page. Click on **accessories** to view and access files.

That's all there is to it!

If you need help, visit:

NewHarbinger.com/accessories

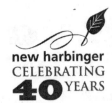

new harbinger
CELEBRATING
40 YEARS